The Native American Herbalist's Bible

3~in~1 Companion to Herbal Medicine

Theory and practice, field book, and herbal remedies.
Everything you need to know from the fields to your
apothecary table

Linda Osceola Naranjo

Disclaimer

The publisher and the author are providing this book and its contents on an "as is" basis and make no representations or warranties of any kind with respect to this book or its contents. The publisher and the author disclaim all such representations and warranties, including but not limited to warranties of healthcare for a particular purpose. In addition, the publisher and the author assume no responsibility for errors, inaccuracies, omissions, or any other inconsistencies herein.

The content of this book is for informational purposes only and is not intended to diagnose, treat, cure, or prevent any condition or disease. You understand that this book is not intended as a substitute for consultation with a licensed practitioner. Please consult with your own physician or healthcare specialist regarding the suggestions and recommendations made in this book. The use of this book implies your acceptance of this disclaimer.

The publisher and the author make no guarantees concerning the level of success you may experience by following the advice and strategies contained in this book, and you accept the risk that results will differ for each individual. The testimonials and examples provided in this book show exceptional results, which may not apply to the average reader, and are not intended to represent or guarantee that you will achieve the same or similar results.

Table of Contents

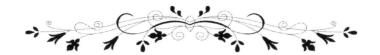

• The Native American Herbalist's Bible 1 •

• The Forgotten Art of The Ancestors of Medicine •

Traditional Herbalism, Modern Methods, and Spiritual Practice
for the Medicine Man of the 21st Century

Linda Osceola Naranjo

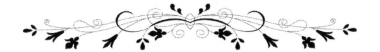

Introduction

"Everything on the earth has a purpose, every disease an herb to cure it, and every person a mission. This is the Indian theory of existence."
Mourning Dove [Christine Quintasket] (1888~1936) Salish

W e live in a country where the cure for virtually any disease and ailment is within our grasp. In our forests, meadows, plains, and gardens grow small, seemingly insignificant flowers and herbs, plants that we don't look twice at, and trees of which we don't even bother to learn the name. Yet, they are the key to a better, healthier, and more sustainable way of life.

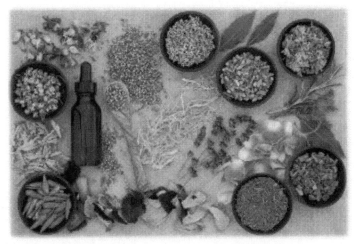

Our forefathers, more attuned with nature that we could ever imagine to be, understood that, and took carefully and sparingly the gifts that Nature offered to heal themselves and grow stronger.
We have lost that knowledge.
Only starting from the 1970s, a renewed interest in botanic medicine has uncovered the depth of the Native American knowledge of plants and their healing powers. The research has not only helped herbalists, but physicians and scientist as well that re-discovered substances that the Native Americans people knew about for hundreds of years.

This book is the unabridged companion to Native American herbs, their traditional and modern use, complete with appropriate doses and usage. The book is completed by a list of simple and effective recipes for the most common ailments.

You don't need to put at risk the delicate natural balance of your body by taking drugs and medications, if an easily available natural solution is just outside your door. Harvest carefully or grow your own herbs, learn to know your body and what works best for you, communicate with the nature surrounding you, and you will in a small way bring back a culture that for too long as been treated as inferior.

This book will teach how to find and treat the herbs the way the native American tribes did: from the forest to your herbalist table, but you will have to find your way to listen to your body and the plants around you.

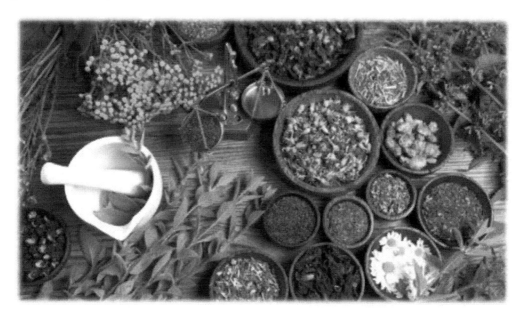

To aid you in your holistic journey, we have decided to divide the book in three volumes. This first volume will give you a full theoretical approach to Native American medicine and the herbal medicines methods and preparations. The second volume is a complete encyclopedia of all the most relevant herbs used in traditional Native American medicine, complete with modern examples, doses, and where to find them, making it a very effective field guide. The third volume is a "recipe book" of sorts: it offers easy herbal solutions to the most common diseases a budding naturopath can encounter. It is meant as a jumping point to find your own way to treat yourself and your fellow man and will come in handy even to the most experienced herbalist.

Native American Medicine and Modern Uses

S ince the 1970s and ever more so today, there is a growing interest in the medicinal uses of herbs and plants for complementary medicine in the U.S. Particularly, both amateur herbalists, professional healers, and physicians, have become aware of the use of herbs by Native American medicine. Many of the botanicals sold as dietary supplements today, have been used for centuries for the same purposes by Native American societies.

However, the commercialized supplements represent only a small fraction of the more the 2500 different plant species that have been discovered and used for their medicinal properties by Native Americans. We shall focus on the most common plants and their properties. This book is meant as an introduction to the native American herbal medicine and this chapter provides a brief explanation to the capital importance of the discoveries made by indigenous inhabitants of the North American continent for modern medicine.

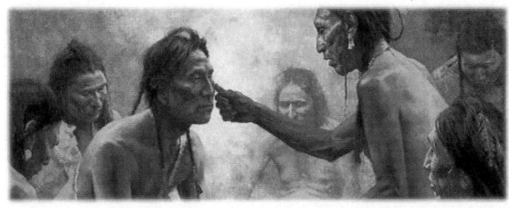

It's an interesting perspective for an amateur or novice herbalist to know the history of the plants he/she wants to use both in traditional medical practices, as well as the current use in modern medicine and drugs. However, if you want to jump right into the herbal dispensatory, you may skip this chapter and read on the basics of herbology in the next chapter and on the plants themselves in the second volume.

Brief introduction on Native American medicine

Native Americans have used herbs medicinally for thousands of years. The first written record of the herbs they used and how they used them begins only with the first contact between Europeans and the tribes, including the Wampanoag, that inhabited the eastern shore of North America. Unfortunately, no written records of herbal use exist before that time to document exactly when they began healing with herbs.

As Europeans immigrated to the New World and as settlers traveled across the plains, the Native Americans taught them how to get well and stay well using nature's medicines. The knowledge the Native Americans have shared with them has given us a rich heritage of healing. In fact, it is believed that at least two hundred of our modern prescription medicines were derived from Native American herbs.

Today, synthetic duplications of natural herbal compounds, as well as naturally grown herbs themselves, account for numerous over-the-counter medicines. As we shall explore in the next subchapter, Native American herbs have been widely commercialized as health supplements, for example.

Our original Americans lived a life of natural dependence in the forests, plains, and coastal regions.

Depending on the area, the Indians used wild species as plant food.

When weather and season permitted a variety of game and fish were utilized as food, clothing, instruments, and decoration.

Berries of all kinds were eagerly gathered in the spring and eaten by everyone as a spring medicine or for specific treatment in hemorrhage and pain due to hemorrhage, high fever, and convalescents, and as a general blood builder.

Cranberries were a favorite autumn food and were also considered as blood and liver boosters. Blackberry roots were used as an astringent.

Nuts were a main source of high nutrition and they used them for making nut bread, crushing them, and adding water for nut milks.

Acorn and dandelion roots were roasted, pounded, and sprinkled over other cooked roots.

Pond lily roots are one of the most widely known food roots on the continent and were eaten from eastern Canada to the Pacific coast.

Milk weed roots were gathered while the dew was still on the leaves and a root sugar prepared from them. The white portions of hardwood ashes were used for salt, also certain leaves.

Apples and other fruits and vegetables were stored in barrels and buried in winter pits. Some were sliced, strung, and dried for later use.

Yucca leaves and Quillaja bark provided soap and shampoo. Although this Indian way of life has vanished, it should be remembered that a considerable number of its elements have been taken over and appropriated by the European colonizers. These included growing of corn, squash, pumpkins, and tobacco. The use of canoes and snowshoes and perhaps still more important and half understood idealization of what is assumed to be an Indian way of life.

The happiest state for a human is when his/her food is also his/her medicine. The Indians at one time were a people of complete accord, for they practiced it daily in many ways.

Native Americans learned which herbs were good for which conditions empirically, often through trial and error.
They tried an herb, and if the patient felt better, then they might use that herb again. A plant's color, shape, odor, and taste also greatly influenced its application. For example, red plants were good for the blood, yellow plants were used to treat jaundice. Plants that looked like the liver were used to treat liver problems. This philosophy of using similar shapes and colors is called the "doctrine of signatures" and is found in the traditional healing art of many cultures. This doctrine is a belief that a plant's physical appearance can reveal its therapeutic benefits. For example, ginseng (Panax quinquefolium) is shaped like male genitalia and was used as an aphrodisiac and to improve sexual potency. The East Coast tribes, including the Delaware, used ginseng to increase male fertility. Sometimes, use of an herb for a particular condition was prompted by a vision or a dream. In fact, a medicine man might experiment with a certain herbal medicine or combination for some time after being given the knowledge in a dream. Another frequently used method of finding herbs was observing the animals to see which herbs they ate.

From the earliest days all Europeans were impressed by the robust stamina of the Indians in every location. The original artist and photographer, as previously mentioned also favors the alert, brave, strong and, in many ethnic groups, handsome Indian in every standard of beauty. Technical study confirms their physical endurance. Archaeology in most cases cannot find any of our modern-day bone deficiency, cavities, arthritis, tuberculosis, etc. Reviewing the scene from another point of view, our studies on the earliest travelers and missionaries also found the Americans very healthy and comparatively 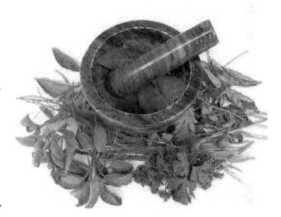 free of disease. From our available sources, we can find only eighty-seven different sicknesses spoken of.

It was uncommon for them to have cancer, TB, or heart conditions, all of which have progressed in our time. The figure of eighty-seven sicknesses is insignificant compared to our modern list of over 30,000 diseases which is growing every day.

Indian women of early history were exceptionally strong. They would often become mother and doctor at the time of delivery and in a few hours resume their daily activity, as their mothers had done before.

In fact, the first Americans were their own physicians in more than one way. Civilization has taught us to build empires for Life Insurance Companies, medical research, welfare, old age organizations, etc.
In comparison, the Indians' protection came from Nature, they learned to treat lives with plant life: medicine from the earth.

After the white man, came they were suddenly introduced to a new way of life which brought them diseases for which they had built no immunity, and thousands died. Self-sufficiency was destroyed as the Indians became dependent on civilized ways.

The Indians were never at a loss to know which plant was best, or the time it should be gathered to be the most efficient cure. They knew how to treat their complaints of physical, surgical and midwifery nature with a skill that surpasses modern medical teachings.

They used vapor baths for many ailments.
Patients were put into sweat lodges of almost stifling amounts of moist heat to eliminate toxic conditions.
Fractured bones were held in splints made of several rods tied together at the ends and covered with leaves and bound with deer skins.
Herb roots were finely pounded and used as a poultice for bad cuts and sprains.
Sore eyes were treated with a wash consisting of an infusion of a certain root.
Cocaine and Novocain come from ingredients found in the coca plant, the nature healer used it to alleviate pain.

The Indian art of healing was ceremonial in nature. To us their rituals seem strange and without meaning, but they knew physical health often failed without the aid of spiritual means. Dancing, chanting, etc., was conducted, according to conditions, or severity of the patient. Today our get-well cards, entertainment troupes, flowers, prayers are less physical but given in the same manner: to support the spirit.
Their health and spiritual source were so closely connected with natural surroundings, they of course were inspired by the significance of nature and to the Sun, Moon, Stars, Rain, Wind, etc., that encouraged it.

Training as an Indian healer began very early. Selection was from the family or from signs of devotion, wisdom, and honesty. It was more than a career, as is of our time, he was elected by ability. Trusted with all secrets, rituals, habits, and legends of their people, while attending all ceremonial celebrations and critical meetings of the people he was at the side of their leader.

The trainee must know and remember the many herbal species, their properties and uses. They knew their limitations and that flowers of the garden are not an agent against the fate of death, but there are flowers for sickness and health and flowers to prolong life. All medical plants in the area were used.
The flora and fauna differed in each locality, but each knew their immediate supply. Modern medicine and natural healing still practice their theory.
Both used strong steam to create perspiration, isolation of communicable diseases, fasting for health, physiological moments, special diets, and of course herbs.
As a healer to all people he was above tribal restriction, he cared for the wounded or needy.
The Indian healer was an artist in the best tradition of Hippocrates' principles.

There are hundreds of Native American herbal cures and more than enough information to substantiate their outstanding healing capabilities. For example, Daniel A. Moerman, ethnobotanist and author of Native American Ethnobotany, documents 24,945 plants used therapeutically by the Native Americans.
In this book I have tried to include those herbs that have historically been used most frequently to treat the conditions listed in the third volume.

In discussing the healing herbs used by the Native Americans, the spiritual beliefs of Native American culture must first be emphasized. These beliefs are tightly, intricately, and unchangeably woven into the tapestry of a Native American's daily life.

It is the combined healing of the spirit, heart, and mind that makes medicine work. For native peoples, the word medicine does not simply describe some physical thing such as a capsule, pill, potion, lotion, or powder (or even surgery); it also speaks of the greater "power" behind the cure.

In addition to their medicinal and food uses, Native Americans have used the plants that grow wild in the fields and forests for weaving, dyeing, basket-making, and for making brushes, ropes, cords, pottery, and decorations. They have used herbs as hunting charms or basket charms and as flavorings and spices.

Herbs were also used in sacred ceremonies, to purify shamans, and to assist in visions and dreams. For example, the great Sioux medicine man and chief, Sitting Bull, had a vision three weeks before the Battle of Little Bighorn that all the white soldiers would fall in defeat and his people would triumph. This is, of course, exactly what happened when Custer and his men met Sitting Bull in battle.

Tobacco was one of the most important herbs for many tribes. It can have both positive and negative effects. According to the Traditional Native American Tobacco (TNAT) Seed Bank and Education Program, "When used improperly, such as when it is smoked in cigarettes, or otherwise ingested in a commercial form, tobacco is a deadly killer. When used properly, in very small amounts in traditional Native American ceremonies and prayer, tobacco (like sacramental wine in a Catholic mass) becomes a positive source of religious power." In addition to tobacco, herbs used in sacred ceremonies and pipe ceremonies include sage, lobelia, gentian, myrtle, magnolia, and slippery elm.

Herbs were of particular benefit in clearing the mind and soul and warding off evil spirits. When used in this way, herbs were often burned in smudges, bundles of herbs that are burned much like incense. Some of the most popular purifying herbs used to please the spirits and the human senses were aromatic, including cedar, juniper, mesquite, pinion, red willow, sage, and sweet grass. Herbs were also smoked for pleasure, as well as for fighting respiratory disorders. A few herbs used for these purposes include angelica, bearberry, corn silk, coltsfoot, dogwood, deer's tongue, mullein, sumac, valerian, and yerba sante.

As mentioned earlier, herbs are used in sweat lodges to detoxify and cleanse the body. Native Americans have also used herbal mixtures in enemas to stimulate the removal of unwanted toxins through perspiration, bowel excretion, urination, or vomiting. In fact, Virgil Vogel, author of American Indian Medicine, notes that American Indians discovered the bulb syringe and the enema tube, using fish and animal bladders plus inserts constructed from reed and small hollow bones.

These Native American techniques were successfully used for centuries and are still in use today. Today, Navajo medicine leaders claim they can even cure people with cancer using routine colon cleansing and fasting, accompanied by sweating.

Enemas used by the Native Americans discarded undesirable toxins trapped in the intestines and worked metaphorically as a way to purify the body in a spiritual sense. Maintenance of a healthy colon is essential for optimal body balance.

The Native Americans have also used herbal laxatives to purge deadly toxins and as a preventive measure against illness. Enemas can be administered at home, or colonic therapy can be performed under the guidance of a trained chiropractor or naturopath.

Although there is a wealth of herbal knowledge present within the culture of American Indians, it is not always easy to encourage Native Americans to part with their herbal secrets. Many feel that Native Americans have been exploited enough through the centuries, and they do not want to perpetuate that exploitation. Others believe that the power of their healing systems might be weakened by sharing them with non-Indians, who might misrepresent the techniques. Many of the sacred songs and healing rituals were passed on during vision quests or initiations into secret societies; so naturally, Native Americans are not comfortable sharing this fragile, sacred information with those who might alter it or abuse it—especially when most who hold the knowledge had to undergo so much in order to attain it.

Fortunately, however, there are those like me, who believe that sharing Native American healing secrets with non-Native Americans is the only way to keep them alive and protect them from extinction. This, then, is my goal: to celebrate the greatness of the Native American herbal healing traditions and to share this information with you so that you can take charge of your life for better health.

The healing properties of herbs

For centuries, Native Americans have used whole herbs for the treatment of disease; and while they knew that the herbs worked, it wasn't always known why. For example, teas of pine needles or rose hips were used to cure colds or flu. As we now know, it was the vitamin C and bioflavonoids in the pine needles and rose hips that possessed the healing action.
Today, science is identifying the healing properties contained in herbs, including vitamins, minerals, enzymes, and phytochemicals.

PHYTOCHEMICALS

Phytochemicals are the naturally occurring chemicals found in plants ("Phyto" means plant). These plant nutrients can be isolated and concentrated from herbs and other plants.
Some phytochemicals are effective as cancer fighters or antioxidants; others lower cholesterol, decrease plaque in the arteries, stimulate immune system function, or stimulate enzyme production. Following are some of the phytochemicals found in many of the herbs used by American Indians over the centuries.

Alkaloids
Alkaloids are found in several plants, including goldenseal. They prevent the overgrowth of yeast in the body, maintaining healthy levels of bacteria in the gastrointestinal and urinary tracts; and they support immune function.

Anthocyanidins
Anthocyanidins are a class of phytochemicals that are found in bilberries, black currants, and raspberries.
They fight free radicals (a by-product of metabolic reactions in the body that can lead to such degenerative illnesses as cardiovascular disease and cancer); reduce blood-vessel plaque formation, maintaining blood flow and reducing the risk for cardiovascular disease; inhibit edema (swelling due to fluid accumulation); fight inflammation; and improve vision.

Chlorophyll

Chlorophyll is found in all green herbs. It fights bacteria, helps in the healing of burns and wounds, and fights cancer. It is also an excellent source of vitamin K.

Diterpenes

Diterpenes are found in many herbs, including rosemary. It is a potent antioxidant, anticancer agent, and anti-liver-toxin agent.

Eleutherosides

Eleutherosides are found in Siberian ginseng. They increase stamina, stimulate appetite, and increase physical and mental vigor. They stimulate metabolism, the immune system, and the central nervous system. Eleutherosides are also helpful in combating some of the problems of menopause, including irregular periods and hot flashes.

Essential Fatty Acids

Essential fatty acids, namely omega-3 and omega-6 fatty acids, are fats that are essential to good health but cannot be made by the body. They maintain the integrity of cell membranes and of myclin sheaths (the protective covering of nerve fibers). They stimulate the production of prostaglandins (hormonelike substances that mediate metabolism, smooth-muscle activity, and nerve transmission, among other functions), lower blood cholesterol levels, and strengthen immunity. They can be found in many herbs, including saw palmetto.

Flavonglycosides

Flavonglycosides are potent antioxidants (fighters of free radicals). They also dilate blood vessels, improving blood flow; improve mental clarity; improve vision and hearing; and help alleviate depression. They are found in Ginkgo biloba.

Gingerols

Gingerols are antioxidants and improve digestion of proteins and fats. They also soothe the stomach and fight liver toxicity and inflammation. They are the active constituents of ginger.

Ginkolic Acid

Ginkolic acid, found in Ginkgo biloba, is yet another antioxidant. It improves circulation and mental clarity, treats depression, and fights cancer.

Glycyrrhizins

Glycyrrhizins, the protective phytochemicals found in licorice, have antiviral, anti-inflammatory, and skin-protective properties. They also inhibit tumor formation.

Hesperidin

Hesperidin, found in milk thistle seeds, is an antioxidant that protects capillaries and strengthens cell membranes. It works well against liver disease and protects against ultraviolet rays.

Hypericin

Hypericin is the active component of St. John's wort. It helps improve mood, possibly by regulating neurotransmitters in the brain.

Isothiocyanates

Isothiocyanates are found in horseradish. They induce the production of protective enzymes and inhibit DNA damage, thereby reducing the risk for breast cancer.

Lactones

Lactones, found in kava kava root, protect the body against cancer by eliminating carcinogens.

Lipoic Acid

Lipoic acid, found in many plant foods, is a potent antioxidant that eliminates heavy metals from the body, protects against cancer and heart disease, normalizes blood-sugar levels, and slows aging. Lipoic acid is a key factor in energy production.

Phenolic Acids

Phenolic acids are antioxidants that inhibit the formation of nitrosamines (cancer-causing agents). They are found in berries, parsley, and all flowering plants.

Phthalides

Phthalides, found in parsley, detoxify carcinogens, and stimulate the production of beneficial enzymes.

Polyacetylenes

Polyacetylenes also are found in parsley. They regulate the production of prostaglandins and protect against carcinogens.

Proanthocyanins

Proanthocyanins, found in elderberry and bilberry, are another class of antioxidants. They protect against cancer, high blood-cholesterol levels, and the influenza virus. They also strengthen blood-vessel walls.

Quercetin

Quercetin is a flavonoid that is widely distributed in the plant kingdom. (Flavonoids are naturally occurring antioxidants found in many fruits, vegetables, and other plants.) Quercetin has antihistamine, anti-inflammatory, and anticancer properties. It also stabilizes cell membranes and reduces capillary fragility.

Rosemarinic Acid

Rosemarinic acid is the active constituent of rosemary. It fights nausea, intestinal gas, and indigestion. It is also effective against headaches.

Salin

Salin, or salicin, is found in white willow bark. It fights inflammation, relieves pain and fever, and fights the influenza virus.

Saponins

Saponins, found in ginseng root, licorice, black cohosh, yucca, and many other herbs, fight cancer formation, enhance wound healing, and reduce cholesterol levels. They have anti-inflammatory, antibacterial, and antifungal properties.

Silymarin

Silymarin is the active constituent of milk thistle. It is an antioxidant and protects the liver.

Tannins

Tannins are widely distributed in plants. They are antioxidants that have antiviral properties and strengthen capillaries. They protect against cancer, heart disease, and asthma.

Terpenes
Terpenes (the common name for monoterpenes) are antioxidants found in Ginkgo biloba.

Triterpenoids
Triterpenoids prevent dental decay and fight ulcers, cancer, and liver toxicity. They are found in licorice root and gotu kola.

ENZYMES
Enzymes are present in all herbs that have not been exposed to high temperatures or to alcohol during preparation. The presence of enzymes is essential in order to activate the phytochemicals and other nutrients in the herbs.
Enzymes also are very important for improving the absorption, action, and bioavailability of these herbs in the body. If enzymes have been destroyed during the processing of the herbal preparation, it is important to take enzyme supplements in addition to the herbs. Enzyme supplements should contain a combination of proteases (enzymes that work on proteins), lipases (break up fats), and amylases (break up carbohydrates).

Native American herbal medicine and modern health supplements

Seven of the most widely sold herbal supplements were used by Native Americans, such as black cohosh (Cimicifuga racemosa), blue cohosh (Caulophyllum thalictroides), elderberry (Sambucus species), and juniper (Juniperus communis). Some pharmaceuticals were originally discovered in the course of investigations of botanicals that were used by Native Americans for medicinal purposes.
Examples are Taxol, obtained from Pacific yew tree (Taxus brevifolia), and etoposide phosphate, a derivative of podophyllotoxin, which is a constituent of May apple or American mandrake.
Both are currently used for the treatment of various diseases. Plants play an important role in the medical practices of many, if not all, Native American peoples. Plants are used not only in the diagnostic and therapeutic process, but also in the physical and ritual purification procedures that commonly precede ceremonies and in the act of healing itself.

The 7 top-selling botanicals in the U.S., their uses by Native Americans, and their current uses

Common name (Latin name)	Family	Native American tribes	Native American indications	Current indications
Ginseng (*Panax quinquefolius*)	Araliaceae	Cherokee, Creek, Delaware, Fox, Houma, Iroquois, Mohegan, Pawnee, Penobscot, Potawatomi	Tonic, expectorant; for fevers, tuberculosis, asthma, and rheumatism; as a strengthener	Immune function and stress
Garlic (*Allium sativum*)	Liliaceae	Cherokee	Stimulant, carminative, diuretic, expectorant, mild cathartic; for scurvy, asthma, and prevention of worms	Cardiovascular health and cholesterol lowering
Echinacea (*Echinacea purpurea, Echinacea angustifolia, Echinacea pallida*)	Asteraceae	Cheyenne, Choctaw, Dakota, Delaware, Fox Kiowa, Montana, Omaha Pawnee, Ponca, Sioux, Winnebago	Pain relief; for coughs and sore throats, fevers, smallpox, mumps, measles, rheumatism, and arthritis; antidote for poisons and venoms	Immune function
Goldenseal (*Hydrastis canadensis*)	Ranunculaceae	Cherokee, Iroquois, Micmac	Tonic; for fever, whooping cough, and pneumonia	Immune function
St John's wort (*Hypericum perforatum*)	Hyperiaceae	Cherokee, Iroquois, Montagnais	For fever, coughs, and bowel complaints	Antidepressant
Evening primrose (*Oenothera biennis*)	Onagraceae	Cherokee, Iroquois, Ojibwa, Potawatomi	For premenstrual and menstrual pain, obesity, and bowel pains	Antioxidant status: premenstrual and menstrual pain
Cranberry (*Vaccinium macrocarpon*)	Ericaceae	Montagnais	For pleurisy	Health of urinary tract

Of the >17000 plant species that constitute the North American flora, > 2500 members of the vascular taxa and > 2800 of all taxa were used—and to some extent continue to be used—for medicinal purposes by various Native American societies. The gathering of information about the use of particular plants as medicine has been in progress for at least a century. The resulting data were compiled in book form in 1986 and, more recently, in an Internet database (http://www.umd.umich.edu/cgi-bin/herb).

Yet, ethnobotanists continue to uncover additional medicinal plants and uses of the plants already included in these databases.

Specific uses of medicinal plants by Native Americans have been reported and, interestingly, the same plant parts were often used by many different tribes in diverse areas of North America.

Analysis of the plants used as medicines by the original North American residents showed that the choice of medicinal botanicals was by no means random, but highly selective, as evidenced by the extensive use of some plant families and the virtual avoidance of others.

Several lines of evidence suggest that Native Americans took botanicals as medicine in the sense that Western science uses that term: for example, Native Americans used different plant parts for the treatment of various ailments, combined several botanicals for specific therapeutic purposes, and recognized toxic plants both as actual poisons and for medicinal purposes.

However, we should also emphasize that a spiritual component is also involved in the use of plants for the treatment of particular symptoms, because it is the power, the "spirit," of the plant that is believed to have the therapeutic effect. For a plant to have "power," certain rules must be observed in collecting the plant.

Even if we could be tempted to ascribe such rites to the religious aspect, rather than the purely therapeutic; it is interesting to note that similar instructions are reported from such geographically and culturally distinct tribes as the Iroquois of the Northeast and the Salishan of the Northwest (Vancouver Island).

In both tribes, the importance of collecting plants in the morning is stressed, tree bark is to be taken from the eastern side of the tree, an offering of tobacco is to be made, and prayers need to be said. Such details regarding the collection procedure or, perhaps more important, the precise plant part used and the method of its preparation, are not always reported.

Despite the availability of many of these botanicals in health food stores and, to an increasing extent, in supermarkets and pharmacies, scientific research regarding efficacy and safety is limited. Most medicinal botanicals have not been investigated to any great extent, and rarely has the focus of such research been specifically on medicinal botanicals used by Native Americans.

Fortunately, however, some of the species used medicinally by Native Americans are also native to other parts of the world (e.g., Sambucus nigra, Sambucus racemosa, and J. communis); others were introduced to European settlers by indigenous North American populations and have subsequently become popular in Europe such as Echinacea species and Lobelia inflata. Intentionally or accidentally, settlers from other continents, in turn, brought some of their native botanicals, resulting in the eventual use of some foreign species by Native Americans (e.g., Urtica dioica and Tanacetum vulgare). For example, U. dioica, stinging nettle is a native of Europe and Asia, its extensive use by Native American societies throughout North America suggests that the plant and its medicinal use spread rapidly after its introduction. Various parts of the stinging nettle were administered externally and internally by numerous Native American societies for a variety of purposes, including as a general tonic (i.e., what we would now consider an immunostimulant) and as a treatment for fevers and rheumatism.

Therefore, what little research exists on species used by original North American inhabitants predominantly comes from other countries where the same species were used, often for the same therapeutic purposes as those reported by Native Americans. Research on botanicals used by indigenous populations has generally been confined to in vitro screenings of individual plants or their constituents for their antibacterial, antiviral, or anti-inflammatory activities. The fact that a botanical was traditionally used for wound healing, fever, infection, edema, or rheumatic disease is taken as an indicator that the plant should be tested for its anti-inflammatory properties.

One of such species that has been studied more thoroughly is Echinacea. E. angustifolia, the narrow-leafed purple coneflower, has long been used by Native 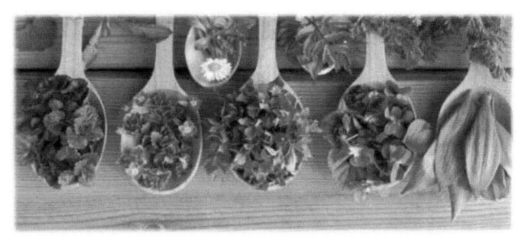 Americans for pain relief and wound treatment, as an antidote against various poisons, and for symptoms associated with the common cold.

It was introduced by Native Americans to European settlers, who subsequently took what they thought was E. angustifolia back to Europe.

It turned out, however, that the species introduced in Europe was E. purpurea, another native American plant used for medicinal purposes by the Choctaw and Delaware.

E. purpurea has since become one of the most popular medicinal botanicals in Europe and the United States. For medicinal purposes, besides E. purpurea and E. angustifolia, a third species, E. pallida, is commonly used.

What the American consumer calls Echinacea can be any one of the 3 above-mentioned species or a combination of 2 or even of all 3 of them, which should of course be indicated on the label.

Furthermore, many Echinacea preparations, including one of the best-known European brands that has been used in numerous studies (Echinacin), are extracts of both root and above-ground parts, whereas in other instances the root alone or the above-ground parts alone are used.

There are substantial differences in the chemical compositions and the biological activities not only between different Echinacea species, but also between their roots and aerial parts.

It is noteworthy that E. purpurea does not contain echinacoside, the substance used frequently for standardizing E. angustifolia and E. pallida extracts. Further differences arise from the extraction procedure. For example, the polysaccharides to which many of the stimulatory effects of Echinacea species on the nonspecific immune system have been attributed are likely to be present in aqueous, but not in alcoholic, extracts.

In addition, in the United States, Echinacea is often sold in combination with goldenseal (Hydrastis canadensis); combinations with other medicinal botanicals are common here and in Europe.

Echinacea is one of 12 commonly used herbs that physicians need to be aware of and knowledgeable about (48). At least 3 different species of Echinacea are sold under that name, yet the literature is often reviewed without regard to what particular species was used. Moreover, differences arising from different extraction procedures, solvents, and plant parts used are ignored, and little distinction is made between data obtained with purified polysaccharides and those obtained with crude extracts.

The consumption of botanical supplements in the United States has been increasing at a rapid rate and this trend is expected to continue. In many cases, the original indications of the putative beneficial effects of botanical supplements appear to have come from their use by Native Americans. Yet, scientific research is still confined to only a handful of the hundreds of substances sold in health food stores.
Not only that, but the few studies on the effects of Native American medicinal botanicals have been conducted in experimental animals, and there are even fewer reports of clinical trials. Nonetheless, what little scientific data have been gathered tend to confirm that many of the plant species contain bioactive constituents that are effective in treating the very ailments for which they were used by Native Americans.

Particularly noteworthy are the indications that some of these medicinal botanicals might be useful in the treatment of chronic inflammatory diseases such as rheumatoid arthritis and SLE. The therapies currently available for both of these conditions are often quite ineffective and are almost invariably accompanied by serious adverse effects. It would, therefore, be highly desirable to find less toxic alternatives, and some medicinal botanicals might be a suitable solution.

Much of the current research appears to focus on attempts to isolate and characterize bioactive principles. However, it should by now be clear that isolated chemical constituents of plant extracts seldom have the same effect as does the complex mixture of bioactive molecules present in whole-plant (or plant part) extracts.
In view of the increasing popularity of botanical supplements and anecdotal and empirical evidence of their uses, new scientific approaches for investigating these supplements need to be developed to allow research to move away from the reductionist principles that have been applied to their study so far.

Sourcing Herbs

Herbalism is not a magical or spiritual practice, it is *science*.
Our ancestors knew a lot more about health and the human body than popular culture gives them credit for, and the practice of herbalism is the collected wisdom of centuries of trial and error. There are still some aspects of herbalism we haven't yet explained with science, but it's not "magic."

Herbalists work with plants because the vitamins, minerals, and organic chemicals that plants create to keep themselves healthy can keep humans healthy, too.

The beneficial properties of herbs as medicines will often depend upon the greenness or ripeness of the plant. The time for cutting and digging is essentghial to the peak susceptibility of its known attributes. Whether it be summer, winter, spring or autumn, the timing must be in accord with the plant's protocol.

For instance, Cascara, or Sacred Bark, after it has been stripped in the proper season from the tree and made into a powder or tincture is more valuable and effective with age. Nettle is a great herb in its earliest stage of growth, but will prove less valuable with age. Another great essential of a plant which is to be selected for its medical qualities is its environment. If indigenous to the locality or country wherein it is found, it is the proper one to select.

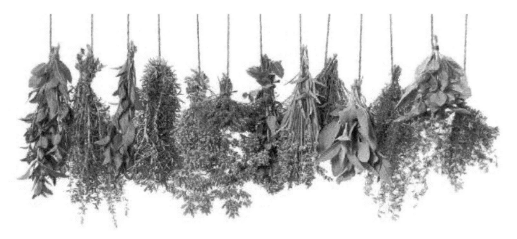

Plants that are introduced from other countries are lessened, or deprived, of their virtues, unless they meet in their new home all the essential conditions possessed in their native place. It must be apparent to all that herbs are liable to suffer from soil, climate, etc., and from these conditions will vary the medical properties attributed to them. When giving a medical herb be informed as to its proper curative effect upon the system.

Because herbs are so complex, it's not accurate to think of them as "weak" or "gentle" drugs. They fit into a complete system of health care that is not the same as the mainstream Western model. The holistic herbal model prioritizes early preventive care, and when illness happens, it focuses on supporting and strengthening the body's own response mechanisms.
Therefore, it is vital to know how to best source and treat these plants, if we want to approach herbalism as a serious practice.

We should not think in terms of "use" in reference to herbs whenever possible. To "use" something implies exploitation.

We should view herbs as teachers, allies, and friends, not mere resources to be exploited, as the Native American tribes did, as the ritualized crafting of the herbs shows.
We don't use our human friends to help us move or plan a party—we work together with them. We feel the same way about plants, and try to reflect that in the way we speak and write about them.

This is one small aspect of an ongoing effort to respect plants as living, independent organisms with their own needs and desires. While plants don't perceive or act on the world the same way we do, they are nevertheless alive and responsive to their environments. (The books What a Plant Knows, by Daniel Chamovitz, and The Hidden Life of Trees, by Peter Wohlleben, are excellent explorations of plant sense and sensitivity.)
It's our responsibility as stewards and caretakers to make sure we take only what we need, minimize waste, and actively restore plant habitats and populations so these beings can continue to share their gifts with us for generations to come. In the spirit of this commitment, we shall heed the example of the Native American spiritual approach to wild foraging.

Native American rituals for wild foraging

It is a spiritual belief that dictates the procedures and ceremonies that are to be followed when herbs and other plants are gathered. Phyllis Hogan, the founder and director of the Arizona Ethnobotanical Research Association, works with a total of sixteen Native American tribes, including the Navajo and Hopi. She is an applied ethnobotanist who has worked in Arizona for nearly thirty years, documenting comparative plant uses among the state's indigenous people.

She also owns the Winter Sun Trading Company, a Flagstaff company specializing in traditional herbs and American Indian art. An expert in the use of southwestern botanicals and the first person to receive the honorary position of practitioner associate in anthropology from North Arizona University, Phyllis was taught by the Navajo to always pick herbs early in the morning and begin by burning juniper, smudging some of the soot on your skin, and praying to the sun deity.

Then, she makes a prayer offering of cornmeal to the plant, telling it her name and that she wants to use the plants to heal. She then asks permission to pick the plant's fellow plants and waits for the plant to give permission. According to Phyllis, "This can be in the form of a vibratory connection between the picker and the plants; perhaps the wind blows or you get an intuitive feeling or hear songs. And if the plant does not give permission, you do not pick that day.

You don't pick the plant you are praying to, because it is your emissary to the plant world. You then give an offering to the earth, then the sky, then the four directions, starting with the east and going clockwise. And also honor the middle. We also put a little cornmeal on our heads. This is a connection to the spirit world and also a sign of purity."

She adds that some plants don't want to come, some pull easily and some won't. It is also important to never take more than you need and always leave at least one-fourth of what's there.

Rare and endangered plants should never be picked, and you should never pick in someone else's picking place. Some areas have been picked for thousands of years by the same clan members. Pickers show respect for the plant world, always wearing nice clothing and jewelry when gathering herbs. This is because they are meeting the deities and want to be recognized as someone of stature. Phyllis's favorite pastime is herb-gathering because she stops thinking of worldly problems during this time.

According to Phyllis, pickers only pick one type of plant per day. "This is because you must take responsibility for the plant and feed it with cornmeal or pollen again, then pray to welcome it." Once the plants are picked they are placed on clean sheets or other cloths and aligned with the herb, roots, leaves, and flowers pointing in the same direction as the other herbs, roots, leaves, and flowers. They are then fed cornmeal once again and welcomed, and told again why they are needed. They are then allowed to rest for a day; only one species of plant is picked a day. Before preparing the herbs, they are again prayed to and thanked for being here. Only then are they prepared into tinctures, extracts, or other forms.

Buying

High-quality herbs are high-quality herbs, regardless of their source. Where you live, that might be a local health food store, a small local farm, or even your neighbor's garden. You may even have an herb shop in your town. You might be surprised to find that your grocery store has good-quality herbs, too, especially those frequently sold as produce. Or you may live somewhere with limited access to herbs, in which case you should find a reputable online retailer.

You'll also find that the price of herbs can vary greatly, depending on where you purchase them. Cheaper is not usually better! Local small producers often have to charge more for their herbs and herbal products, but the quality is also often much higher.

Experiment with small batches first, so you learn which producers have the best quality; that will help you know whether it's worth the money.

There are a few things to keep in mind when sourcing herbs: soil quality, growing practices, and how the herbs are dried or processed.

If the soil where the herbs are grown is contaminated with heavy metals or other pollution, this is likely to be in the plant matter. It's important to know where the herbs were grown, so you can determine whether the soil was clean. This can be a problem for herbs grown anywhere, but especially those grown in places that don't have regulations about soil pollution. Some larger herb retailers, such as Mountain Rose Herbs, test their herbs to make sure they are free of soil-based contamination.

You might be disinclined to purchase herbs grown in urban farms, but don't write them off: Talk to the producers and ask about their soil. Most urban farms bring in clean soil and use water filtration to make sure their produce is safe.

Growing practices are also important. How were insects managed? What kind of fertilizer was used? Were the herbs grown in a greenhouse or outdoors? Were they grown hydroponically or in soil? All these things have pros and cons, but the bottom line is the result: If the herbs have vibrant color and strong aromas and flavors, then the quality is good.

The drying and processing step can be tricky, too: High-quality herbs can be ruined if they're dried at too high a temperature or stored improperly. You'll know this is the case if there is significant browning in the dried herbs. This is the same browning you would see on a living plant that had a brown, dried leaf—it looks un-vital. Let's use St. John's wort as an example: This plant should have some brown when it's dried, but its brown color is a deep-red mahogany. That's very different from the brown-black color of basil leaves that have gone bad in your refrigerator. The latter is the one to avoid.

The bottom line is, know who you're buying your herbs from. Ask about their growing practices, about the soil and water, and about their processing practices. Not only does this help you make good choices, but it also helps build community between the people who grow our herbs (and food) and those of us who consume them. When we understand more about where our herbs come from, we value them, our farmers, and our environment more.

Wild Crafting

Although it's alluring to think about hiking out into wild places and harvesting your own herbs, most times, the best advice we can give is, actually, not to do this.
There are some very abundant and fairly safe herbs to wildcraft, but overharvesting is a serious problem for our wild herbs, and when so many can be organically cultivated, it is really much better to do that instead of taking plants from the wild.

Some herbs should be avoided altogether, because they are at risk of extinction from overharvesting and habitat destruction. Many plants, especially woodland plants, require healthy forests to grow in and can't be cultivated. Some of these plants, such as goldenseal, osha, and black or blue cohosh, are very popular and are still being sold. However, just like vegetables, there are many herbs with similar qualities, so there's no need to purchase these at-risk plants. You can learn more about at-risk herbs and those that should be avoided at the United Plant Savers website, unitedplantsavers.org.
Some popular herbs should also be avoided because their sale exploits the people and communities they come from. In general, when there's a new trendy "superfood" from some far-off place, we avoid it. Maca is an example: Touted as a plant that will give you more energy, and that is also quite delicious, people flocked to it. But maca is a subsistence food for the indigenous Peruvians living at high altitudes, and the more that industrialized nations purchase, the more expensive it becomes: Local people can no longer afford to eat it. Issues like this are complicated, but when it comes to exotic superfoods, it's always good to remember we have our own superfoods right here. Plants such as cranberries, nettle, and dandelion leaves don't have the exotic appeal, but they're every bit as super!

However, it is very rewarding to find wild plants and work with them, so here are some guidelines for doing so safely—for you, for the plants, and for the ecosystem they are a part of!

WILDCRAFTING ETHICS AND GUIDELINES
Prepared by the Rocky Mountain Herbalists' Coalition

Wildcrafting
1. Never gather an endangered or threatened species. Check your local herbarium or botanical garden for a list of these plants. You may also contact the American Herbalist Guild for a national listing: AHG, Box 1683, Soquel, CA 95073.
2. I.D. positively before harvesting. Use identification keys and voucher specimens.
3. Ask permission and give thanks, acknowledge connection with all life, share your appreciation.
4. Leave mature and seed-producing plants—grandparent plants—within the stand and at the top of a hill to seed downslope. Work your way up.
5. If unsure, harvest no more than ten percent native whole plant and root, and thirty percent naturalized plant species or native leaves and flowers. Gather only from abundant stands. Harvest conservatively to insure maintenance and well-being of plant communities.

Site Selection

1. Obtaining permission: On BLM land, a free use permit may be obtained for a minimal charge if you are collecting small amounts. Both the U.S. Forest Service and BLM will tell you there is no picking (a) in or near campgrounds or picnic areas; (b) any closer than 200 feet from trails; and (c) on the roadsides.
2. Stay away from downwind pollution, roadsides (at least 50 feet), high-tension electric wires (may cause mutations), fertilizers in lawns and public parks, downstream from mining or agribusiness, around parking lots, and possible sprayed areas. Some BLM and Forest Service districts use routine spraying. This applies to private land as well, and you may need to ask about herbicides and pesticides.
3. Use discretion with fragile environments—one irresponsible wildcrafter can severely alter a rocky hillside or streamside ecosystem.

Gardening and Propagation Techniques

1. Using proper wildcrafting techniques will insure minimal impact, increase harvest yields, and continue to provide plant food for wildlife. Do not harvest the same stand year after year, but tend the area as necessary. "Gardening" techniques that apply include thinning, root division, top pinching, and preserving a wide selection of grandparent plants to seed and guard young plants.
2. Be aware of erosion factors. If digging roots, replant or scatter seeds, and cover holes. Be mindful of hillside stands, replace foliage and dirt around harvested areas. Gathering foliage from nearby harvested plants and spreading it around may be necessary. Wearing hard-soled shoes may cause delicate hillside ecosystems irreparable damage.
3. If harvesting leaf, don't pull the roots. Flower pruning of certain plants will increase root yields as well as foliage.
4. Make seasonal observations on wildcrafted areas. Be mindful of your harvested stands and check different growth cycles. This will determine your real impact on the ecosystem. (One experienced wildcrafter in the northwest has observed that a healthy population will increase about 30% a year until it reaches stasis. Anything less than this could be considered degenerative.)

Suggested Gathering Times

1. Aerial or above ground parts: Mornings between 6 and 10 a.m., just before they wilt in the sun. If harvesting leaf, many are best just before flowering. Harvest most flowers just as they are beginning to bloom—you should be able to see the color of the bud. The traditional moon phase for harvesting aerial parts is near or during the full moon.
2. Roots: Harvest after seeding; if possible, in the early morning before the sun hits. Biennials: Harvest in the autumn of the first year or the spring of the second year. The traditional phase is the new moon.
3. Barks: Harvest in the spring or fall. Never strip. Take the whole tree. Tree thinning is appropriate in dense populations, but always leave the healthiest looking trees. If you take from the small branches only, be aware of potentially leaving the tree vulnerable to fungal rot. For many barks, the inner bark, or cambium, is the most active. Leave short trunks for pollarding, and low stumps for coppicing. This will provide an ongoing harvest. The traditional phase for barks is the three-quarter waning moon.
4. Saps and Pitches: Harvest in late winter or early spring.

5. Seed and Fruit: Harvest when mature, with some exceptions such as citrus, unripe scarlet bean pods, etc.

Growing

No matter how urban your surroundings, you can grow your own herbs. There are many herbs that will grow happily in a pot near a sunny window—you don't even need a yard! If you've never grown any kind of plant before, or if you've ever described yourself as having a "brown thumb," don't worry: Growing plants is just like any other thing you want to do. Spend a little time on it each day, and soon enough it will seem easy.

Some herbs are definitely easier to grow than others. Mint, catnip, sage, and yarrow are easy ones to start with and can be found as seedlings or seeds at your local garden center. Mint and catnip are very easy to grow indoors as well. All are perfectly happy to live in pots if you don't have a yard or if you don't have safe soil to grow in. You can have your soil tested with your local Extension Office—they'll send you a testing kit and provide results about soil safety as well as tips about the best type of fertilizer to use with the type of soil you have—all for about $10. Your local Extension Office also offers classes and advice about gardening in your area, as well as many other services, for free or at a low cost. (You can search "county extension office" to find the one near you).

Most of the herbs you will end up using are worth growing yourself, although proper wild crafting is the best choice, it is quite time-consuming.

Here are 11 plants you might consider growing yourself. They are mostly quite easy to grow, especially from a plant rather than seeds, if you don't have a green thumb or time to grow your plants from seeds or seedlings. They are all quite common and inexpensive.

1.**Garlic**: infection fighter, stimulant
2.**Rosemary**: cancer-fighting antioxidants, stimulant
3.**Basil**: antioxidants, infection fighter
4.**Mint**: stimulant, digestive
5.**Lemon balm**: relaxing tonic for mild depression, irritability, anxiety
6.**Fennel**: anti-inflammatory, analgesic, appetite stimulant, anti-flatulent
7.**Lovage**: respiratory and digestive tonic, anti-bronchitis
8.**Oregano**: antiseptic, anti-flatulent, stimulate bile and stomach acid, anti-asthmatic
9.**Cilantro** (coriander): to treat flatulence, bloating and cramps; breath sweetener
10.**Horseradish**: perspirant, stimulant
11.**Thyme**: tea for preventing altitude sickness, antiseptic, inhalant (anti-asthmatic), stimulant

Just like with herbalism, the best way to get started growing herbs is just to start! Buy a seedling, put it in a pot with some good dirt and a little water, and check on it every day. Plants are living beings, and you'll learn to "hear" your plant's communication in the same way you learn to understand what your cat or dog is trying to tell you!

Preparing Herbs

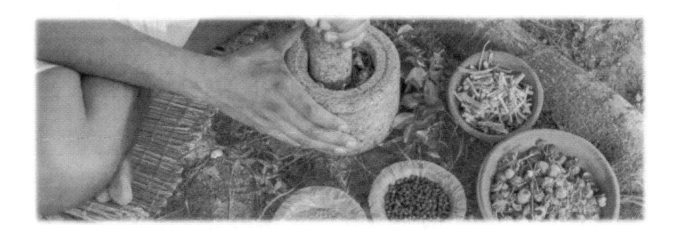

Herbal preparations

Modern technology provides superior ways of distilling, extracting, purifying, and standardizing herbal extracts that are beyond the scope of this book.
Nevertheless, so that you may use this guide more effectively, we will go over some simple preparations for the complete beginners.

Tea: Prepare tea (also known as an infusion or tisane) by pouring hot water (just off the boil) over fresh or dried herbs. Typically, the soft parts (leaves and flowering parts) of the plant are infused. Examples: green teas, black teas, herbal teas. Amount: One teaspoon dried herb to 1 cup of water; 4 teaspoons of fresh herb to 1 cup of water.

Decoction: A liquid made by simmering or boiling herbs in water. Decoctions pull water-soluble chemistry from the hard parts of the plant: the stems, seeds, bark, and roots. Example: Garlic soup. Amount: Simmer one teaspoon dried herb to 1 cup of water; 4 teaspoons fresh herb to 1 cup of water. Simmer for at least 5 minutes, strain and use.

Percolation: Percolation is a process like making coffee: Water or alcohol is dripped through a damp mass of powdered herb. Example: Dripping hot water or alcohol through cayenne powder. Put a drop to your lips…. Zowee! Amount: Drip 100 milliliters of liquid through 10 grams dried herb; and then repeat the process over and over to increase concentration.

Tincture: Chopped herbs, blended in alcohol. Other chemicals can be used in place of alcohol, such as apple cider vinegar or glycerin. The maceration (blending of the chopped herb) can be accomplished in a blender. Example: Dilute a volume 190 proof alcohol (Everclear 95% alcohol) with an equal amount of water to get approximately 50 percent alcohol.

Then chop fresh cut Echinacea flowers into small pieces, place in a blender, and cover with 50 percent alcohol, then macerate.

Let the maceration rest in the refrigerator for four hours, then strain and bottle. Amount: When making a tincture with a dry herb, typically a 1:5 ratio is used—that is, 1 ounce of the dried herb is macerated and blended with 5 ounces of 50 percent (100 proof) alcohol. With fresh herbs a 1:2 ration is often used—1 gram to every cubic centimeter of 50 percent (100 proof) alcohol.

Double Extraction: For a double extraction, first fill a container such as a 1-quart canning jar (or like container) with a cup of macerated (ground) Echinacea leaves and roots (or other plant material to be extracted). Completely cover the maceration with 8 ounces of 50 percent diluted Everclear (add an equal volume of water to an equal volume of Everclear to get 50% alcohol concentration). Then cover. Allow blend to sit for a few days (up to 2 weeks) in a darkened cupboard or refrigerator, shaking twice a day. Strain off the liquid—a pair of pantyhose is an effective strainer—and then run it through an unbleached coffee filter. Squeeze out the remains in the filter when it has stopped dripping. You now have a "single extraction." Now take the Echinacea mash (marc), cover it with water, and simmer for thirty minutes to make a decoction, adding water as necessary. Strain and then blend the decoction with the tincture, making a stronger "double extraction." To maintain an alcohol concentration of at least 25 percent (50 proof) add no more water to the second extraction than the original amount of the 50% alcohol used to make the initial extraction. That is, if you poured 10 ounces of 50% alcohol over the herb in the first step, do not add more than 10 ounces of water for the second extraction.

Fomentation: Prepare a decoction or infusion of herbs (see decoction and infusion above), then dip a cotton cloth into the preparation and wrap the warm, wet cloth around an injury. Example: Dip a cloth in a mild cayenne extraction and apply it to an arthritic joint. (Note: This application will redden the skin and may irritate.) Amount: Enough to cover area to be treated.

Poultice: Pound and macerate fresh herbs and apply the moist herb mass directly over a body part. Example: Put a warm, wet, and pounded mass of plantain over a pus-filled wound. Amount: Large enough amount to cover area to be treated.

Powder: Powders are prepared by drying and finely grinding the herb, then loading the powder into 00 capsules (1gram capsule, or 1,000 mg). Example: Many over-the-counter dried herbs are powders sold in capsules. Amount: A typical dose may be one 500- to 1,000-milligram capsule.

Oils and salves: These can be prepared with dried or fresh herbs. First the herb is cooked in oil to extract the active principle, then the oil is thickened or hardened with beeswax. Example: The aerial parts (flowers, leaves, and stems) of yarrow are covered with oil and simmered then blended with warm beeswax. The blend is cooled, and the resulting salve is applied as a wound treatment. Amount: With yarrow I lightly pack a pan with fresh leaves and flowers and cover with olive oil or lard (studies suggest lard is better absorbed through human skin than plant oils).

Essential tools

It doesn't take fancy equipment or rare, expensive ingredients to make high-quality herbal preparations. Most of what you'll need is probably already in your kitchen.

Mason jars. These are the herbalist's best friend. Because they're made of heat-resistant glass, you can pour boiling water right into them to make tea. They're also handy for making tinctures, storing herbs, and more. Quart- and pint-size jars are the most versatile, though for storing dry herbs you may want larger jars. Many store-bought foods (sauerkraut, salsa, etc.) come in mason jars—just hand wash or run them through the dishwasher and dry to reuse them.

Wire mesh strainers. For straining tea or pressing out tinctures, you'll want strainers of various sizes. Start with a few single-mug strainers for making one cup of tea at a time, as well as a larger, bowl-size strainer for filtering larger amounts of herb-infused liquids.

Cheesecloth. This is handy not only for straining and squeezing herbs you've infused into liquid but also for wrapping the herbs in a poultice.

Measuring cups and spoons. Cup, tablespoon, and teaspoon measures are all helpful, as well as some graduated measuring cups with pour spouts, which allow you to measure down to a quarter ounce.

Funnels. A set of small funnels is extremely helpful for getting tinctures and other liquids into bottles with small openings.

Bottles. For storing tinctures long term, amber or blue glass bottles are best. The "Boston round" type is a favorite for tinctures and other liquid remedies, but any shape will do. Get in the habit of saving and reusing any colored glass bottles you come across—there are a number of kombucha brands that come in amber glass, for instance.

One- and two-fluid-ounce bottles are most convenient for dose bottles, while storage bottles are usually 4 to 12 fluid ounces. For storage, use plain bottle caps, but you'll need dropper tops for dose bottles.

Labels. Label your remedies as soon as you make them. Address labels are sufficient for most purposes—even a bit of masking tape will do in a pinch.

Blender. For mixing lotions, breaking down bulky fresh plant matter, and other purposes, a standard kitchen blender will serve just fine.

Useful instruments

These tools make it easier to integrate herbs into your life, especially if you have a busy schedule, but they're not as necessary as those preceding.

French press. This is our favorite tool for making herbal infusions. It allows the herb material to float freely in the water and exposes a lot of surface area for extraction (you just press down to easily dispense filtered tea), and it is simple to clean.

Thermos. When traveling or bringing your tea to work, a good thermos is an asset. There are versions that include a filter built directly into the lid, so you can put the herbs and water directly into the thermos together from the start.

Press pot. This is an insulated pot with a lever you press to dispense. People usually put coffee or strained tea into these, though we've found you can usually get away with putting herbs directly into the pot, pouring in boiling water, and letting it infuse in there. It'll stay hot all day, and you just dispense it by the cup. (Hold a little mesh strainer under the spout to catch any herb bits that pass through the tube.)

Herb grinder. A simple, small coffee grinder served us well for many years, but if you plan to make a lot of herb powders you may want a larger, dedicated machine.

Ingredients

Herbs and water alone will serve for a great many remedies, but some preparations require additional ingredients.

Alcohol. Tinctures are mixtures of herb extracts and alcohol. We usually use vodka or brandy.

Apple cider vinegar. Always use this, rather than distilled white vinegar, for herb-infused vinegars, oxymels (a blend of vinegar and honey), and topical applications.

Honey. Choose local honey whenever possible, unprocessed/unfiltered if you can get it. Beware that some big-brand honeys have been found to be contaminated or even contain high fructose corn syrup. Liquid honey is easiest to use in herbal honey infusions, while thicker honey can be more manageable for first aid and wound care.

Oils. You can use olive oil for most purposes, though in some instances you'll want a lighter oil, such as grapeseed or almond, or a thicker oil such as shea butter or cocoa butter. You can even use animal-derived oils, such as lard, tallow, or lanolin.

Beeswax. Salves require wax to thicken them. You can buy beeswax in rounds or chunks and cut it down for each use. You can also buy beeswax pellets, which can be easier to work with.

Witch hazel extract. Look for a witch hazel extract made without alcohol, as this is most versatile—especially for first aid or wound care.

Rose water. Traditionally used for skin care, though also as a food ingredient. Rose water from the "ethnic foods" section of the grocery store is just as good as the higher-priced stuff in the health and beauty aisle.

Sea salt and Epsom salts. For baths and soaks as well as nasal sprays and gargles, a bit of salt improves the medicine.

Gelatin capsules. The "00" size is most frequently used when working with herbal powders to make homemade herb capsules.

Safety Tips

Label everything. If you don't know what you're taking, you can't be sure it's safe. Include details about all the ingredients in the remedy, as well as the date it was made.

Start small. Begin with small test batches and small doses when working with a new remedy. You can always scale up or take more later, but if an herb or preparation doesn't agree with you, it's best to discover that with a small amount.

Be cautious with pharmaceuticals. Herbs and pharmaceutical drugs (including both prescription and over-the-counter medications) can interact in many ways. Sometimes this is beneficial—positive herb-drug interactions may allow someone to reduce the dose of a drug or minimize its side effects—but it is a complicated subject and should be handled very carefully. We identify the major interactions to watch for in the notes that accompany each remedy, but it's always best to consult with a practicing herbalist familiar with this topic, or your health care provider, especially if multiple drugs are taken simultaneously.

Use your senses. Look at the herbs you're working with, and your finished product. Check for mold in your jar of infused oil, check for bits of packaging material in your shipment of dried herbs. Smell and taste your herbs and remedies to get a sense of their potency, and dose accordingly.

Make only what you need. If you get great results from a particular remedy and you want to have it on hand every day, great—go for it. But no one needs a gallon of nasal spray solution, and it'll go bad before you even get around to using it. Make only those remedies you need, and only as much as you need.

Begin with what's abundant. You will most likely start with herbs that are highly prevalent in the wild or grown commercially on a large scale. As you branch out into working with other plants, keep your focus on those that are local to you, and neither at risk nor endangered. Don't be tricked into thinking a rare, exotic herb will be the only one to solve your problem.

Get the herb to the tissue. Herbs need to be in contact with the affected tissue to help it. We can't always just drink some herbal tea and get good results. Choose a delivery method that helps your herbs get where they need to act.
A few examples: If you're working with a respiratory problem, go with a steam; if you've got something on the skin, apply a soak or poultice; if it's trouble in the lower intestine, swallow some powder so it's intact when it gets down there.

Four essential methods for the budding herbalist

Now that you have a general idea of how to prepare herbal remedies, let's take an in-depth look at the four methods traditionally used by native American tribes.

Plants are generally taken as medicines in four ways (though this is by no means exclusive): in water as **infusions or decoctions**; as **tinctures** from extended immersion in an alcohol and water combination; as **salves** from transferring the power of the herb to an oil base; and in an **unchanged state** either by chewing or eating the root, or grinding the plant and taking it directly or in capsule form.

When changing the plant into another form for use as medicine, the healer said prayers for each stage of the progress.
They believed that sitting with the plant and calling on its spirit with ceremony and prayer would bring it into aliveness and turn it into true medicine.

Feel free to give thanks to the Creator, or Nature, and respect the spiritual bond between men and Nature. Even if you don't believe, it will help you reach with time a deeper more meaningful connection with the plants and therefore make your treatments more effective. After all, putting into more "scientific terms" when you demonstrate deep care and attention to your work, you are less likely to make mistake and use the gifts that you were given with more acute focus.

Making Infusions and Decoctions

An infusion is made by immersing an herb in either cold or hot (not boiling) water.

The water should be the purest you can find, not tap water. Water from rain, healthy wells or springs, or distilled water is best.

Herbs that have strong volatile oils (those that have a strong fragrance like an essential oil or perfume) are best infused in cold water. Other herbs do well in warm water.

They should be left for a period of time, from fifteen minutes to overnight, depending on the herb, to allow the water to absorb the essential elements of the herb.

Glass or earthenware vessels are best for making infusions and decoctions.

Quart or pint canning jars are very good as they will not break from heat, and the screw cap keeps the nutrients from floating away in the steam.

Main'gans
An Example of a Hot Infusion

This infusion is used for its general nutritive properties, especially for women in menopause.

1. Mix together one pound each of dried, cut, and sifted nettles, oat-straw, red clover, alfalfa, horsetail, and spearmint.
2. Put one cup of the mixture in a quart container, fill with hot water and screw on the lid. Leave overnight. In the morning strain the mixture to remove all the herbs and drink the mixture throughout the next two days.
3. Do not keep infusions longer than two days as they begin to go bad.

The rule-of-thumb is to take 16 ounces (two cups) per day of an infusion for someone weighing 130 to 160 pounds.

In general, use the following guidelines to make infusions with hot water:

Leaves: one ounce per quart of water, four hours in hot water, tightly covered. Tougher leaves require longer steeping.

Flowers: one ounce per quart of water, two hours in hot water. More fragile flowers require less time.

Seeds: one ounce per pint of water, thirty minutes in hot water. More fragrant seeds such as fennel need less time (fifteen minutes), rose hips longer (three to four hours).

Barks and roots: one ounce per pint of water, eight hours in hot water. Though some barks such as slippery elm need less (one to two hours).

Cold infusions are preferable for herbs, which perform differently in cold and hot water.

Yarrow, for instance, can be quite bitter when prepared in hot water but is not bitter when prepared in cold water. The aromatic components of yarrow, and their corresponding antispasmodic properties, are soluble in cold water while the bitter components of the herb are not.

Cold infusions are prepared in the same manner as hot infusions but each herb will need to be immersed a period of time specific to itself. This can only be learned over time though many herbal books on the market can give guidance (see reference section for suggestions).

Decoctions, prepared with boiling water, can be much more potent than infusions. The general method is to take one ounce of herb in three cups of water and boil steadily until the liquid is reduced by half.

Use only a stainless steel or glass container, never aluminum. The dosages can range from a tablespoon to a cup depending on the plant used. Decoctions should be kept only a maximum of two days, refrigerated.

Tincturing Herbs

A tincture for internal use is made by immersing a fresh or dried plant in either straight alcohol or an alcohol and water mixture.
Plants, when fresh, naturally contain a certain percentage of water. A fresh plant is placed in 190-proof alcohol (95% alcohol), one part of plant per two parts of alcohol.

For example, if you had three ounces (dry measure) of fresh yarrow it would be placed in a jar with six ounces (liquid measure) of 190-proof alcohol.
Mason jars are very good for this. The top is screwed on and the tincture is left for two weeks out of the sun.
At the end of that time it is decanted and the herb squeezed in a cloth to remove as much liquid as possible. Alcohol pulls out of a plant all the water it contains.
The resulting tincture will be a mix of both water and alcohol.

With fresh plants I do not cut or chop them into tiny pieces though many herbalists do so. They feel that the more surface area that is exposed to the alcohol, the stronger the tincture. In my own work, the herbs prefer to be left whole.

I rarely tincture roots fresh. When I do, I chop them into smaller pieces. Above-ground plant material I always leave as whole as I can when tincturing. Each person must find what works best.

Plants, as they dry, lose their natural moisture content.
Tables are available on the moisture content of many medicinal plants. A good one is offered by Michael Moore through his Southwest School of Botanical Medicine.

Some plants like myrrh gum contain virtually none and others, like mint, contain a lot of water. When making a tincture of a dried plant you add back into the mixture the amount of water that was present in the plant when it was fresh.

Generally, dried plants are tinctured at a five-to-one ratio; that is, five parts liquid to one part dried herb.
For example, osha root contains 30% water by weight. If you have ten ounces of powdered osha root you would add to it fifty ounces of liquid, 35 ounces of 95% alcohol and 15 ounces water.

Dried herbs are generally powdered as finely as possible, often in a blender. It is best to store them whole until they are needed. Again, the tincture is left for two weeks and then decanted, and the liquid squeezed out of the herbal material.

With fresh plants you can generally get out about as much as you put in. With dried material, especially roots, you get out as much as you can.
Amber jars are quite useful for tincture storage as they protect the integrity of the tincture from the chemical breakdown that can occur from sunlight. So protected, the tinctures can last many years.
Herbal tinctures can then be combined together (though a certain few do not combine well) for dispensing. Because of their long keeping quality and ease of dispensing many herbalists prefer tinctures.

A Combination Tincture Formula for Upset Stomach
1. Ten milliliters each of yarrow, poleo mint (or peppermint), and betony.
2. Place in a one-ounce amber bottle with dropper.
3. Take 1/3 to 1/2 dropper as needed.

This mixture will usually quiet an upset stomach or nausea in seconds.

Making Oil Infusions for Salves

The first part of making a salve is to transfer the medicinal properties of the plant to an oil base. Then the oil is made thick and moderately hard by the addition of beeswax.

1. To make an oil infusion of **dried herbs** grind the herbs you wish to use into as fine a powder as possible.
2. Place the ground herbs in a glass baking dish and cover with oil. Olive oil is a good choice.
3. Stir the herbs to make sure they are well saturated with oil then add just enough oil to cover them by 1/2 to 1/4 inch.
4. Cook them in the oven on low heat for eight hours (overnight). Some herbalists prefer to cook the herbs as long as ten days at 100 degrees.
5. When ready, strain the oil out of the herbs by pressing in a strong cloth with a good weave.

1. To make an oil infusion from **fresh herbs** place the herbs in a mason jar and cover them with just enough oil to make sure that no part of the plant is exposed to air.

2. Let sit in the sun for two weeks.
3. Then press the herbs through a cloth. Let the decanted oil sit.
4. After a day the water, naturally present in the herbs, will settle to the bottom.
5. Pour off the oil and discard the water.

Some herbalists prefer to start the oil infusion by letting the herb sit for 24 hours in just a bit of alcohol that has been poured over the leaves. They then add the oil and allow to stand for two weeks. The water and alcohol remain behind when the oil is poured off.

Making Salves

Put the oil infusion into a glass or stainless-steel cooking pan. Heat gently on top of the stove.
Add chopped beeswax to the warmed oil, usually 2 ounces per cup of oil.
Many people like the beeswax grated but I just break it up in a number of pieces and put it in. It melts fine that way.
When the beeswax is melted, place a few drops on a small plate and let cool. Touch it—if too soft add more wax; if too hard add a bit more oil. Pour into a jar and let harden uncovered. Use the following formula for a good wound salve:

1. Add oil to heavy pot. Do not use aluminum or cast iron. Glass or stain less steel is best.
2. Grind all herbs into fine powder, or as close as you can get.
3. Add herbs to oil.
4. Cook overnight in oven with low setting (150 to 200 degrees).
5. Take out and let cool, then press herbs in cloth to extract all oil.
6. Clean pot; return oil to pot and reheat slowly on stovetop.
7. Measure out about 4 ounces of beeswax (generally 2 ounces of wax to every pint of oil).
8. Add vitamin E, about 1/4 teaspoonful, and stir in.
9. Pour into salve containers and label.
10. You may add essential oil if you want to give a fragrance to your salve.

Some wounds do not respond well to a wet dressing like a salve. In that case I use the powdered herbs directly on the wound. The herbs used in the wound-salve formula, when ground into a fine powder, stop bleeding and facilitate rapid healing while preventing infection. After the wound has begun to heal, wound salve continues that process.

The comfrey root facilitates rapid cellular healing and wound closure with less chance of a scar. Echinacea, usnea, chaparral, and osha provide antibacterial, antifungal, and antiviral properties. Burdock is an excellent skin remedy and cranesbill stops bleeding.

Using Whole Herbs
The same herbs used in the wound salve are excellent when placed directly on a wound. They are powdered as finely as possible, combined together, lightly dusted on the wound. The fine powder helps reduce friction against the wound that sometimes occurs from larger, rougher grinding and it can be added to socks and shoes to treat athlete's foot.
Many herbs can be eaten when needed. Osha is a prime example and can be used for sore throats and upper respiratory infections of both viral and bacterial origin. It is very strong and a little is eaten when necessary. Sometimes a combination of both whole herbs and tinctured herbs works well.

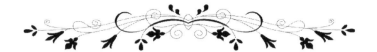

Storing Herbs

If you don't dry and store your herbs properly, they will quickly use their effects.
Fresh herbs can lose intensity very quickly, so if you don't need to use them immediately, dry them immediately after you've sourced them.

To dry herbs, separate the leaves from the stems and spread them in free, single layers on a spotless, leveled surface. Bulkier plants might be dangled from a line in a dry zone, for example, a warm storm cellar or attic. Flies and different bugs might be attracted by your hanging herbs, so you might need to cover them with a cheesecloth.

The time required for drying depends both on the herb and the earth in which it's being dried. Since herbs lose their strength so rapidly, the shorter the drying time frame the better.
For most herbs, it takes about seven days. An herb is adequately dry when it despite everything has a smell yet is sufficiently dry to break. On the off chance that it disintegrates totally when you handle it, you dried it excessively long.

Roots, which ought to be completely washed before drying, take more time to dry than leaves and flowers—for the most part around three weeks.

Although you may have seen pictures of old homesteads with dried herbs hanging from the rafters, these days we have better storage methods to ensure your herbs stay fresh and last a long time.

The universal standard for storing basically any herbal product is mason jars.
Whether dried herbs, tinctures, salves, elixirs—likely as not, herbalists put it in a mason jar. They come in all sizes; they're widely available, airtight, and inexpensive. The only thing they lack is color: dark-colored glass, such as amber or cobalt, prevents light from affecting the quality of the product you're storing. But those containers are more expensive, and, realistically, clear glass is fine as long as it's not in direct sunlight.

If stored in glass with a tight-fitting lid, you can expect dried herbs to last 1 to 5 years, and tinctures might last as long as 10 years.

Oils and salves have a shorter shelf life, because oils go rancid eventually—they may only last 6 months to 1 year.

Lotions have the shortest shelf life, because when you mix oil and water, you have a perfect medium for mold. Lotions may only last 1 to 3 months, but you can extend their life by refrigerating them.

The best way to detect if dried herbs or herbal products are still good is to use your senses: If it still smells strongly of the herb, if it still has bright vibrant color, if it still has potent flavor, it's still good.

SUMMARY

Drying

1. Dry most plants in shaded, well ventilated areas, avoid wire screens and newspaper print. Research which plants dry better in the sun.

2. Don't wash leaf or flowers. Shake them to get bugs and dust off. If the quantities are manageable, tie bundles at the base of the stems in diameters of 1 1/2 inches or less. They may also be scattered loosely on screens to dry.

3. Barks: Scrape off the outer bark if appropriate. This is called Tossing.

4. Roots: Lay them out or string. Rinsing usually will not remove soil particles. A pressure hose is often required as well as hand brushing, especially with clay. Cut lengthwise for large heavy roots without aromatic properties.

5. All plant parts are dry when brittle. Pinch the lower part of hanging plants. Cut large sample root in half to see if center is dry.

Storage

1. Avoid light and excessive heat that could destroy aromatic properties and other valuable constituents. When totally dry, food grade plastic bags or fiber barrels or other containers that omit oxygen and moisture are desirable to preserve quality and potency as long as possible.

2. Label with dates and location.

3. Broken or crushed herbs lose their value more rapidly than whole, uncut herbs.

Sacred Medicine

I have left the most complicated matter for the last chapter of this first volume.
Up until now I have spoken of Native American Medicine as matter-of-factly, scientifically-proven therapies and treatment.
I talked about how herbal medicine was incorporated in pioneer and modern medicine and how we can utilize its wisdom to this day as herbalists and healers. This was by design, this book after all is meant for beginners and specialists alike, and spirituality cannot be forced upon anybody. One should come to it to his/her own accord. However, one should not forget that tribal medicine was not simply the decoction of herbs.

Although this book is about herbal healing, herbs are only one part of the overall Native American philosophy of health. At the heart of Native American healing is a trust and belief in a higher power—the Great Spirit, the Creator—and the role He plays in our everyday lives. Each tribe or nation has its own name for this Great Spirit. The Arapaho call It "Man Above," the Pawnees refer to It as "Ti-rá-wa," the Crows speak of It as "First Maker," and the Sioux call It "The Great Spirit" or "Mystery."

The animals, the plants, water . . . everything in nature are gifts entrusted to us by our Creator. According to American Indians, if properly cared for, these gifts will feed us, clothe and shelter us, care for us when we are sick or injured, and keep us healthy. But these gifts bring responsibilities to care for and to respect nature and the universe and to use these gifts only as needed. People are an essential part of the universe, but only a part of a whole, lovingly fashioned by the Creator. Almost every Native American culture believes that everything— every animal, living creature, plant, rock, tree, mountain, and even water—has a soul. Therefore, all of nature must be treated with respect and honored.

As I've mentioned, they didn't interpret medicine as a reaction to a symptom. The medicine man was a deeply spiritual figure within the community and the healing was ceremonial as well as factual.

Nowadays, ceremony may be self-derived, it may come from vision, it may be given by a teacher, it may be cultural. But from all sources it has the same underlying root. It is a process in which the human capacity for sacred feeling and reverence is given form and expression. One tells the Earth, one tells Creator, what is felt and thought through specific actions and movements and intentions. This underlying intention held within the ceremonialist is given outward expression in ceremonial form. And in the process humans, the spirit world, the different elements of Earth are bound together in a living fabric that is alive, vital, and new.

It has long been known among indigenous cultures that when people forget their place in the web of life without periodically renewing connection with the sacred, illness and disharmony follows.

John Seed notes that the Hopi, living in the longest inhabited settlements in North America, still don ceremonial masks and perform community ritual designed to restore connection to the Earth. He makes the point that this connection must be frequently reexperienced during ritual if it is not to be lost. This propensity to lose connection is probably a normal and natural part of our human makeup. Connection must be renewed through ceremony over and over again.

Many ceremonies are simple, for often it is not the form of the ceremony that is important but its intention and meaning. It is a simple thing to thank Creator for life each morning, to ask for the help of the plant relations, to smudge with sage.

There have been many primary ceremonies and rituals developed to help people once again be in balance with the web of life. Among the North American indigenous cultures some of these are the sweat lodge, the sacred pipe, vision quest, and the medicine wheel. In working with sacred plant medicine, I have found two of these to be of special power and benefit—the sacred pipe and the medicine wheel.

The sacred pipe ceremony shows how detailed and sophisticated ceremony can be when filled with the directed intention of spirit. Further the pipe, like many Asian ceremonial processes, is specifically focused on the act of uniting Heaven, Earth, and Man.

This unique joining has particular relevance to sacred plant medicine and a great deal can be learned from it.

Finally, the use of the pipe was moderately common among practitioners of sacred plant medicine.

The medicine wheel incorporates an essential element of sacred plant medicine, the indigenous understanding that all of life is a circle, that each element of the life web sits together in a council of life, and that human beings travel around a great wheel as they progress through life.

Thus, the medicine wheel has particular relevance because it is a highly developed expression of the Earth-centered experience. It incorporates the belief that there are unique and specific stages of human development that transcend psychology and environment, and that plants have a specific place in helping at certain stages of travel around the wheel. Finally, herbs sometimes contain within themselves the power of a specific direction, and awareness of this power when working with plants can be of special benefit during healing ceremonies.

Each of these ceremonies can utilize smudging: the sacred pipe always, the medicine wheel sometimes.

So, before I go into detail on these two ceremonies, let's see what smudging is all about.

Smudging

Smudging is the act of burning an herb and "washing" one's self, the other participants, and the plants or ceremonial tools in its smoke. The act of smudging demarcates the ceremonial event in time, saying that from this point on what we do is sacred. Historically, one of four herbs have been used for smudging: cedar, sweetgrass, sage, or wormwood.

When smudging, the dried herb is placed in a bowl or other container and ignited. The flame is then extinguished, allowing the herb to smolder. The smoke that rises is then fanned on the object or person being smudged, using one's hands or a feather.

The herbs traditionally used for smudging are thought, in all cultures in which they are used, to clear negative influences and restore balance.

The Sacred Pipe

The American Indian ceremonial pipe has been in use for centuries. The earliest pipes that have been found are simple tubes discovered in prehistoric mounds in Ohio. They are made of clay and alabaster. The earliest long stemmed pipes had bowls made in the shape of animal heads.

The use of ceremonial pipes spread along the Mississippi River and into the lakes and eastern plains around the 11th century. One of the first tribes observed by Europeans to use the pipe were the MicMac of Nova Scotia. The pipes have been used in holy ceremonies by Earth-peoples for at least a thousand years.

—JOHN FREESOUL

Most indigenous peoples of North America who use the pipe have legends of its creation or appearance in their culture. Some tribes received it as a gift from another tribe, others received it from holy people or supernatural beings who were sent by Creator to bring it to humans. This gift of the pipe by the intervention of Creator through a sacred being or prophet is akin to the tablets given to Moses in Hebrew tradition, or the appearance of Christ in Christian tradition.

Each part of the pipe represents certain things.

The bowl is the female, the stem the male. The flesh and blood the bowl, the bones the stem. The bowl the Earth mother, the stem Father Sky. The channel through the pipe stem and bowl represents the direct connection between all things and Spirit, the straight and narrow path each human walks to be in relation with Spirit. Thus, when the pipe is joined, all these things are joined as one. Duality is gone.

The tobacco that is smoked in the pipe is made from a variety of plants. There is often tobacco (Nicotiana), mullein (Verbascum), uva-ursi (Arctostaphylos), sage (Artemisia), raspberry (Rubus), red willow (Salix), and sometimes many other herbs.

Whenever possible, the pipe carrier must pick the herbs. The plants should be picked in a specific sacred manner and prepared as smoke mixture by the pipe carrier. Prayers of thanks are offered to the plants who give themselves up to be smoked.

When smoking the pipe, pinches of tobacco mixture are offered to the four directions, the plant kingdoms, the animal kingdoms, the elementals, Great Spirit, Creator, the Earth, the sky, humans, sun, moon, all those in Spirit, the rocks of the Earth, and sometimes many more. In this way, when the pipe is smoked, the whole universe participates.

With each puff of smoke a prayer is offered to be carried up to Creator, Great Spirit. The pipe is used in prayer for whatever is needed. There are some guidelines in addressing the integrity of these prayers—that the prayers honor all life, human and nonhuman, and the continuing existence of all relations, not just human. In this way the pipe is a major Earth-centered tool because it belongs to all life, not just humans. It represents and speaks with the life essence in all things. In this way, the pipe carrier is not the owner of the pipe but its keeper. The pipe carrier is a spokesperson for all life and the life force of creation.

There are specific pipe ceremonies, depending on the lineage and culture of the pipe carrier, and the visions that have given rise to specific pipe ceremonies number in the hundreds or, perhaps, thousands.

The pipe can be used for communion with Spirit, help during difficult times, or for healing the sick. How it can be used in these instances varies tremendously depending on the need or use of the moment. Pipes are made from many materials besides the well-known pipestone; any soft stone will do. Alabaster and soapstone, for instance, are often used. The stems can be made of any wood that feels right. If one is called to the pipe, the correct form will soon present itself.

As the pipe carrier engages in the pipe ceremony over time, a deep relationship with the pipe is established. Eventually the pipe "awakens" and comes alive. An awakened pipe is a channel between the pipe carrier (the human community) and Spirit. Just as there is a spirit and soul in all things so, too, is there one in the pipe.
The pipe carrier establishes relationship with the spirit of the pipe and through it acts as a sacred intermediary for the human community, the Earth, and for all life.

Frances Densmore makes a reference to this event in her article "The Belief of the Indian in a Connection Between Song and the Supernatural." She notes:
On one occasion the writer was questioning Lone Man, a trusted Sioux informant and singer, concerning information received from a pipe. He was asked whether a spirit had entered into the pipe and gave the information. He replied that this was not the case, saying that under certain conditions a pipe might "become sacred" and speak to the Indian.

This living spirit of the pipe is and should be consciously evoked and related with by the pipe carrier when working with the pipe in ceremony.
Almost all Earth-centered practitioners have some physical object of the Earth that is used for ceremonial purposes. These objects become a focus for communion with Spirit and an honoring of the soul and spirit essence in all creation. They often play a special part in Earth relationship and rites of passage for humans. It is a tool for balancing between the worlds and developing depth of Spirit for those on the Earth-centered path.

Each part of the pipe ceremony represents communion with a sacred archetype of the universe. As years are spent in this communion one comes to understand these archetypes and to be in personal relationship with them. Through them one approaches closer to Creator and one's own true nature. The special power of the sacred, which comes from this process, can be evoked to help one's self, friends, family, and community during troubled times.

When people work with sacred plant medicine they are consciously evoking the power of Heaven and Earth by calling on Creator in their prayers. Within the body of the practitioner of sacred plant medicine, the two are united in balance and sacred power is evoked when the plants are called on to become medicine. When one uses the pipe this process is enhanced.

The pipe is akin to many martial art forms that have their origins in Asia. These martial arts have at their center the act of joining Heaven and Earth in the body of the practitioner. This act is a unique one and central to any deep knowledge of sacred plant medicine. In the following detailed account of a generic pipe ceremony, the specific mindset necessary to each ceremonial stage is discussed. Each act deepens the joining of Heaven and Earth and then goes on from there to direct intention toward some expected outcome. This process is central to all forms of ceremony.

To truly understand ceremony and enter into that world, one should come to understand that certain states of mind, of power, exist for which there are few words in the English language. But indigenous tribes, closely connected to the sacred as a part of their cultural life, had well-developed terms for these things. This is especially true of the pipe.

Terminology of the Sacred

In all tribes, each had a specific term that was used to refer to the sacred. The term among the Sioux was *wakan*, among the Ojibwa, *manido*, among the Omaha, *wakanda*, among the Mandan, *ho'pinis*. These are similar to the Asian *tao*.

The act of limiting those terms to mean "sacred" is somewhat incorrect, however. It means much more than that.
The word refers to the sacred center of all things from which all things have come.

So, using Sioux terminology, and quoting Joseph Epes Brown, the degree of wakan a thing possesses *"is in proportion to the ability of the object or act to reflect most directly the principle or principles that are in Wakan-Tanka, the Great Spirit, who is One."*

The commonness of this concept among indigenous cultures in the Americas indicates a general sensitivity to perceiving manifestations of the sacred and a refined capacity to distinguish the degree of sacredness a thing possessed. As this characteristic was so fundamental to all things in indigenous life, understanding of the pipe or any other sacred object or ceremony would be impossible without it. Within each origin tale of the appearance of the pipe to native peoples, these particular terminologies are present, the meaning of which is culturally implied; thus, it is imperative to understand that which is not said as well as that which is said.

The Ceremony of the Sacred Pipe

The pipe as a sacred tool combines the most powerful elements of two processes. First it is equivalent to the Buddhist meditation process of working with a *koan*. *Koans* are statements designed to force one beyond the rational meaning of words into an awareness of a higher truth.

The pipe, when worked with devoutly can, like a *koan*, stimulate one beyond this everyday normal reality into an awareness and understanding of deeper sacred truths. Second, the pipe is an act in which the inherent duality of the universe is made one.

Each act in the pipe ceremony represents a specific sacred meaning. In other words, there is an underlying discrete and specific spiritual meaning that is evoked at that moment in the pipe ceremony. Though there are differing elements in pipe ceremonies, depending on the lineage and type of pipe being smoked, generally all pipe ceremonies are identical in essence.

Besides the pipe (bowl and stem) there are usually a number of other objects that go up to make a pipe bundle. There is the smoking mixture in its own container and a pipe tamper— usually a stick that is narrower at one end, used to pack the pipe before it is lit and during the smoking itself—and matches. There is also smudge, usually sage or wormwood; a container in which to carry it; a smudge bowl; and often a feather or bird wing to be used to waft the smoke onto the objects being smudged. There is usually an altar cloth or small rug on which everything is placed, and a container in which all these things may be kept. Then there are any other sacred objects that may be important to the pipe carrier and all of these, together, are carried within a ceremonial pipe bundle.

When the pipe bundle is unpacked the altar cloth is laid down and the objects are laid out. Smudge is lit and everything is smudged, beginning with the people involved in the ceremony—the pipe carrier first. The pipe is usually smudged last—the stem first and then the bowl. When the stem and bowl are smudged many pipe carriers pass them across the smudge bowl north to south then west to east. The stem first and then the bowl are held, their opening to the lips, and smudge drawn through them so that they are purified inside and out. In this beginning element of the ceremony the mind has a chance to quiet itself, the participants to take on the proper attitudes and states of mind. This signals that what is to follow is a sacred thing, set off from what has gone before.

The next step is the joining of the stem and bowl. The bowl is held in the left hand, the stem in the right and both are held up to Creator and permission to smoke is requested. This is the first act that is koan-like in its nature. The pipe carrier acts as an intermediary for the manifestation of the sacred. It is through the carrier's training, directed intention, and sensitivity that the ceremony evokes all the power of the holy, that it is truly wakan. At this point one listens for permission to be granted; if it is, then, and only then, are the bowl and stem joined. At the moment of unity, the duality of the universe is made one. This act is central to the nature and purpose of the pipe. It is through this joining and the participatory smoking of the pipe that divisions, human and nonhuman, between people and cultures, between secular and sacred are transcended. All things become one.

The next step is the filling of the pipe. The bowl rests on the ground, the stem in the lap. Generally four pinches of tobacco are used to fill the bowl. With each pinch some portion of the web of life is invited to come into the circle and into the pipe. All life is brought into the process.

A pinch of tobacco (smoking mixture) is taken between the thumb and first two fingers in the right hand, held up to Creator, and a prayer is said.

For example:
Creator, Grandmother Earth, all my relations
all the Spirits of this place
I ask that You come and join us now
There is a place for You in this pipe
A second pinch is taken and held up to Creator, the prayer continuing:
All the green relations
spirits of tree, and osha, and all the green growing things
I ask that You join us now
There is a place for You in this pipe
A third pinch is taken and held up to Creator, and again one prays:
All the animal relations
the two-leggeds, the four-leggeds, the wingeds, the
swimmers and crawlers
I ask that You join us now
There is a place for You in this pipe
And finally, a fourth pinch is taken:
I call on the powers of the four directions, the
stone people, fire, water, and air
All the star relations, all those who have walked this
path before us
I ask that you join us now
There is a place for you in this pipe

As each pinch is taken and as each part of the life web is invited to come and join in the pipe ceremony, the pipe carrier is intently focused on the underlying meaning that is being evoked. The participation of these other members of our world is actual and literal. One must be able to feel them come and take a seat in the council circle of the pipe. Often many years of work are necessary to truly evoke these powers, to feel them actually come and take their place, to create dialogue and communication.

In the fourth step, prayers are placed in the pipe. If others are participating in the ceremony the pipe is passed to the left. The person takes the pipe and holds it, bowl in left hand, stem in right. Anything that person desires to pray for is voiced. For example: if one needs help with a certain thing, for others or oneself, to offer thanks for the help of Creator, to voice a pain that is carried, thanks for a joy felt, anything, it is offered at this time. The pipe is passed around the circle until it comes back to the carrier.

The fifth step is the lighting of the pipe. The pipe is lit, puffed vigorously until it is going well, then it is held up, stem first, for Creator to smoke. This is another portion of the ceremony that works with underlying meaning. The pipe carrier works with personal sensitivity, humility, and intention until the time when one can feel Creator actually come and smoke the pipe. After Creator smokes, the stem is lowered and offered to Grandmother Earth. When Grandmother Earth smokes the pipe it is offered to the Four Directions, one after another, until each one has smoked. Then, and only then, does a person smoke the pipe.

The sixth step is the smoking of the pipe. In this process, a person engages in a deeply interactive process with Creator. The smoke is drawn into the mouth, then into the lungs, and released into the air, whereupon it rises up. The prayers in the pipe take on a visible form. Further, they blend with the body; a portion of this sacred prayer remains in the body and a portion of the body intermingles with the prayer. Then the prayer leaves the body and rises up to Creator, becoming a part of all the universe. In this process the individual becomes joined with all things. The process of smoking is continued until all the tobacco in the pipe is gone.

When the pipe is empty the carrier holds it up and thanks Creator and all things for the pipe:
Creator, I thank you for the gift of this pipe
and as I (we) go forward from one day to the next
from one pipe to the next
I (we) say "Yes, yes, yes, yes"
A-ho!

Then finally, the pipe is taken apart, cleaned, and put away.

The Medicine Wheel

Is not the south the source of life, and does not the flowering stick truly come from there? And does not man advance from there toward the setting sun of his life? Then does he not approach the colder north where the white hairs are? And then does he not arrive, if he lives, at the source of light and understanding, which is the east? Then does he not return to where he began, to his second childhood, there to give back his life to all life, and his flesh to the earth whence it came? The more you think about this, the more meaning you will see in it.
—BLACK ELK

There are few permanent shrines in Earth-centered spiritual lineages. Two of these are the medicine wheel and the sweat lodge. Though the sacred circle is present in all cultures the medicine wheel, a specialized form of the sacred circle, is not. Some version of the sweat lodge is present on all continents and all cultures.

From William K. Powers' YUWIPI: Vision and Experience in Oglala Ritual, published in 1982 by the University of Nebraska Press.

Architecturally, the only permanent shrine in Oglala religion is the sweat lodge. It stands, sometimes wavering in the wind, in sharp contrast to the countless Christian churches that dot the reservation—little frame boxes with identical steeples and church bells that look as if they had all been constructed by a mission construction company. All are painted a sacramental white and have blue- or green-shingled roofs. It is as if they had come off an assembly line, just the way federally funded housing projects deliver prefabricated homes intact to the owner's land.
The sweat lodge is a perfect symbol for the Oglala religion; when not in use the structures look rather pitiful: a dome made of willow saplings stuck into the ground, bent over, and tied in place with cloth strips or rope. There is something exceedingly profane about them when not in use, in contrast to the white man's shrines and churches, which are perpetually sacred, set off from the rest of society in a feeble attempt to separate religion from the culture's social,

political, and economic institutions. The sweat lodge reflects the Oglala principle of austerity and simplicity: the entire universe is a cathedral: everything is permanently sacred unless desecrated by human foibles that cause disharmony between humans and the rest of nature. At this time a special ritual is required to reinstate a balance among all living things, and only then are special places like the sweat lodge temporally and spatially separated from the rest of the mundane world; it is only during the ritual itself that special rules of conduct are in force and require different behavior toward nature.

When not in use, the sweat lodge becomes a playground for children, who dodge in and out of the framework, stepping into the central hole where the heated stones are placed during the ritual. It is a stopping place for multitudes of dogs, who lift their legs and declare the sacred saplings, placed there in honor of the various aspects of Wakantanka, their special territory. It is a meeting place for ants, spiders, grasshoppers, and flies seeking refuge from predatory birds who alight on the willow frame during their morning feeding. The sweat lodge is often invaded by a recalcitrant cow or a frightened horse, and it tolerates all these intrusions, along with the constant battering of the wind against its desiccated skeleton. It is partly this tolerance that makes the sweat lodge potentially sacred: like humans, it is subject to the whims of nature and must abide by its relentless impositions.

Like the sweat lodge, the medicine wheel is usually an unimpressive structure. Most are simple circles of stones laid in a pattern on the ground. They are overgrown easily and, if left untended, cannot be found in a few years. But they have an ancient history, from Stonehenge to the 20,000 or so examples on this North American continent. They serve as a pattern for focusing awareness and as a way of relating to all living things.

In the past, when people would encounter a place on the Earth where the sacred was manifesting itself, where hierophany was strong, they would often construct a circle of stones to mark it. In effect, the stone circle said, "This place is sacred. When you enter this place you enter a sacred space and time." In time, more stones would be added to the circle, rising as walls and more clearly defining sacred space. In some cultures, these would be roofed over and become churches. Sometimes, like the ancient shrine of The Mother of the Hunt in Bandolier National Monument in New Mexico, it would become a low wall. In other places there would be only a circle of stones.

The medicine wheel represents the circle of all life. When you sit in the wheel and evoke the sacred, all life comes to sit in council. The human, only one member of the web of life, can use the ceremony of the wheel to restore contact with all the relations of life. The animal relations, plant relations, stone people, spirit relations, all things come to sit in council. Our connections with the world are thus restored and the healing of the Earth begins anew.

The wheel of life, the medicine wheel, is a map for everything in the universe, a blueprint of the web of life. As Black Elk said, this wheel exists in all things. Within each of us, too, the medicine wheel exists as our inner council.

A human cannot sit in relationship with all life if the life inside is in disarray and disharmony. It is important to understand how the medicine wheel exists inside you and to work to establish harmony in all its parts. From this starting place you can then move outward to larger and larger external circles, finally encompassing all of the universe.

The Medicine Wheel inside You

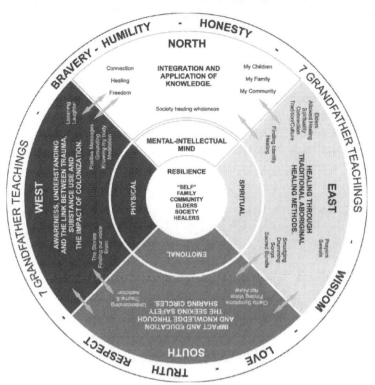

To begin working with the medicine wheel inside you, with your inner council, find a place where you will not be interrupted and that is comfortable to sit. Take a couple of deep breaths and let yourself relax.

When you are ready close your eyes and imagine yourself walking along a path in a meadow. It is a peaceful meadow and you can hear the sounds of the birds and the wind in the grasses. As you walk you come to a small rise; you follow it up. As you clear the top you can see ahead of you a small building; the door is open. You approach it and go in. It is one large room. In the center of the room is a large oval table with chairs around it, many chairs. There may be people, animals, or other beings sitting in the chairs and some chairs may be empty. There is a place for you. You sit down and look around the table. These are the members of your inner council, the parts of yourself that are often not attended to in daily life. There is the child, the wise parent, the one who says "no" to everything, the warrior, the sage, and many more. There are rarely fewer than fifteen members of the inner council. Talk to them and make their acquaintance.

Over time it is important that you are in good relationship with them all, that not one of them is outside the circle inside you. This may take a long time. Some of them may be angry with you for not paying attention to them for so long. If you work at it you can come to joint agreement about all actions you take in your life. Then no part of you will be holding out, no part unenrolled in your choices, no sullen part of you hating what you are doing. This results in a powerful and strong wholeness (from the word holy) in yourself and in your life and actions. It takes some dedication to achieve it. I usually recommend that people speak with their inner council each morning for at least one year. It usually takes that long to really get to know them all and reestablish good relations.

From this exercise you can see how the medicine wheel can be applied externally as well. Instead of parts of ourselves taking places around the wheel, members of community or family or the life web take places around the wheel. These other beings or people are then worked with in the same way as we work with our internal parts are to establish relationship and balance and harmony.

Working with the inner council is a crucial one in sacred plant medicine. If one travels into sacred domains one is working with the substance of reality, that which makes up who we think we are, what we think others and the world are, and that which really is. This process is a difficult one in that travelers may spend many years examining and restructuring deep elements of their personality. This is necessary because their unconscious parts affect all other acts that take place in their lives. If one fears heights, then one avoids them or feels great fear when height is encountered. Even the thought of a great height can induce fear. To gain power one must of necessity understand the root of this fear and transcend it.

When working with plant medicines, it is often the case that in the beginning it is very hard to distinguish between projected feelings and true information coming from the plant. Intense work over many years with the inner council helps identify what is coming from what source, a skill that is essential in this field. Further, many sacred states are fearful or unsettling. It is necessary to be able to hold one's balance at all times. Strong bonds with one's inner council allow that balance to exist, and further, the members of the inner council act as allies during times of spiritual intensity. In addition, members of one's inner council communicate in their own way with the plants, and richer, more varied learnings are available when one has established the bonds of friendship with one's self.

Creating a Medicine Wheel

The ceremony of building a medicine wheel restores all life by reenacting an ancient rite of making sacred a circle, a holy place to remind all to live in good relationship with all life in this universe. This simple circle of stones becomes a vortex of energy as all life forces are honored in ceremony and join the wheel of life. The restoration and building of holy places in balance and harmony with all life is returning the gift of life given to us by Creator and creation. The wheel is a mandala for the dance of life, the unending spiral of interdependence.

Besides the demarcation of sacred space, the stones also represent the members of the Earth community who come to sit in common council. In the circle of stones there are four gates, each corresponding to a direction of the compass—north, south, east, west. In the center of the wheel is a larger stone that represents Spirit, which is at the center of all things. Each of the directions represents a specific archetype and is often a focus of how that archetype manifests itself in human life.

Though there are minor differences between people who use the medicine wheel as a sacred rite, the underlying archetypes and patterns are essentially identical.

The south represents the beginning of life, childhood, the time when spring returns and the new grasses grow. It is the time of hope and the surging vitality of life. The time of renewal and rebirth. At this time one is in contact with caretakers, such as parents or other nurturing beings. One receives.

The west is the time of adolescence when childhood is beginning to pass and one begins to struggle with the demons in one's own soul. This is the time when the warrior within awakens, the time when one goes to the "looks-within-place," that place within all of us where we examine who and why we are. It is a time of going into the dark and finding one's balance and strength; the time when one searches for the unique identity that is one's own; when one strives to identify the meaning and reasons for one's life. At this time people struggle with the stripping away of that which has become unimportant. This destructuring process is often painful and the warrior within each of us awakens to help solve the problems facing us at these times. The end result is personal strength, balance, the capacity to be a warrior if needed, the ability to go into the dark and be unafraid.

From there one moves to the north. The north is the time of middle age, of maintaining the status quo. On the shoulders of those in the north rest the old ones, the young ones sit upon their laps. They are the ones who do the work to help the human world continue. This is the time of caretaking and giving, the time when one can put aside one's self and pay attention to others. The first time of maturity.

From there one moves to the east. The east is the time of enlightenment and old age, when wisdom is the order of the day. The things of youth have been given up and one is concerned about the passing on of wisdom to the young. One begins to have a deeper relationship with the Spirit world and is getting ready to pass over. These patterns occur over and over again in all life, with each thing a human does.

To make a wheel, you must first choose the place for it to be. A quiet corner of your yard is good. Even a quiet place apart in your home would work, though it is better to have it outdoors. When you decide on a place, one that feels good, say prayers to this place, smudge with sage, and declare your intention to create a wheel. Then it is time to find the stones. Go out to places where you feel good, wild places, and saying prayers for help, begin looking for stones: eight larger stones for the gates to each direction, a minimum of four stones between each of the gates, and a large central stone representing the source of all things. Sun Bear's books on the medicine wheel, especially Dreaming with the Wheel, offer other approaches to creating a wheel and go into great detail.

Smudge each stone you find, and say prayers, leave a tobacco offering in exchange for taking it.

Take it to the place where you are constructing the wheel. When you have all the stones ready, with ceremony, begin the wheel. Ask each stone where it wishes to be placed, then place it there. When the wheel is finished you may add more stones to it later.

Like the sacred pipe, each element of the medicine wheel represents a specific meaning. Over time, just like the pipe, it is important to sit in meditation with these different aspects of the wheel and come to understand their deeper significance and be in relationship with them. Once such a level of understanding is developed the particular meanings of the wheel can be evoked for aid in healing and desired directed outcomes.

In working with plants, one becomes aware that there are certain similarities between specific plants and the different sacred powers that are represented in various aspects of the wheel. These plants, in other words, seem to hold within themselves the power of the south or the north. Some seem to hold the whole of the medicine wheel within them.
So, when one works with these plants, not only the medicinal power of the plant is evoked but also the power of the specific direction that the plant holds within it. Understanding this can aid when helping a person with a specific plant medicine.

Some people struggle with leaving the south, the place of childhood. They resist moving into the west, the place of young adulthood. They resist the development of warrior spirit that is integral to the west; resist encountering the darkness that all humans must face in life; resist learning how to carry their own sword.
For someone struggling with this, it can be beneficial to give a plant that is of the west to help the person move around the wheel in that direction.

As another example, for persons who have been stressed out for a long time, who have been overly responsible and parental and lost touch with their childlikeness, one may decide to give them an herb of the south to help them remember this aspect of themselves, to help restore balance.

As you come to feel the essence of the directions, you will be able to identify them in the plants you come to know and use for medicine.

Sweat Lodge Ceremony

For centuries, Native Americans have used sweat lodges and fasting as ways to benefit from the healing properties of detoxification. Of all the purification ceremonies in North America, the sweat lodge ceremony is the most widespread. The Lakota call the ceremony inikagapi, and the Chippewa called the sweat bath ritual a madodoson. The Apache called the sweat lodge itself taachi, while the Cheyenne called it vonhäom. Similar in action to a sauna, the sweat lodge's heat and moisture help detoxify the body—mentally, physically, and spiritually. The smoke in the lodge and the ceremonial rituals conducted there all contribute to the native healing process.

Sweat lodges have several health benefits:

- In the sweat lodge, healing can begin for many physical or emotional disorders. It is an opportunity to pray, speak, and ask for forgiveness from the Creator, as well as from other people who have been previously hurt.
- The cleansing heat increases body temperature, thereby increasing the body's enzymatic activity. This increased activity helps the body destroy viruses and bacteria and stimulates immune function. The famous Greek physician Hippocrates once said, "Give me a fever and I can cure any disease." Increased temperatures help the body to practically burn away bacterial and viral agents and illnesses.
- Physically, sweating helps detoxify the body by opening any clogged pores and allowing elimination of internal toxins, heavy metals, excessive urea, and metabolic by-products.
- As the body's temperature rises, endocrine glandular function is stimulated. This helps to cleanse the body and improve body function.
- The heat of the sweat lodge dilates the large blood vessels and capillaries which, in turn, stimulates increased blood flow to the skin and increases the rate at which the body's organs are flushed of toxins.
- The moist air of the sweat lodge improves lung function. Clogged respiratory passages are dilated, giving relief from minor respiratory problems and colds. Caution: Individuals with major respiratory problems and pneumonia should not use the sweat lodge.
- Hot water and steam created by pouring water over the rocks result in negative ion release. Positive ions are associated with tension and fatigue, as well as allergies, rheumatism, arthritis, insomnia, and asthma.
- Sweat lodges can improve metabolic function. By removing toxins and other waste products, as well as improving circulation, the digestion, absorption, and utilization of herbs and other nutrients can be improved.
- The sweat lodge can be a cleansing and regenerative experience, much like a rebirth. In his book Sweat, Mikkel Aaland observes, "The warm, dark, moist ambiance inside a sweat bath is easily likened to a womb, even the womb of Mother Earth, Herself."

Sweat lodges can be many different sizes and shapes and are constructed using materials found in the local environment. For example, tribes of the Southwest built circular subterranean sweat lodges in which individuals descended a ladder to the underground structure, which was encased in bedrock. Other tribes used mud, wood, or animal skins to build sweat lodges. Cedar planks were used in the far Northwest; buffalo skins covered the Plains Indians' sweat lodges, while skins or birch bark might cover frames made from willow poles in the Northeast.

In the Southeast, sweat lodges might be dug into a hillside or built up into earth mounds. The polar Inuit Indians even used igloos as sweat lodges.

The sweat lodge typically holds ten to fifteen people comfortably and is light-tight to ensure that they are in total darkness. Usually, hot rocks are heated on a fire and then brought into the sweat lodge. The ceremony leader then pours water onto the rocks to produce steam to encourage sweating and cleansing and to stimulate spiritual healing. Prayers are then recited, songs are sung, and the spirits are called into the lodge in an effort to purify the participants. The door is rarely opened during a ceremony, because the heat and dark are important to help the participants focus on what they are doing.

Do ~It ~Yourself Sweat Lodge

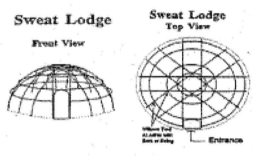

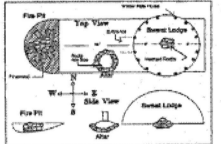

If a sweat lodge is not available, a sauna, such as those found at any health club, makes a good substitute. Or you can build your own sweat lodge. Follow the American Indian's example and use materials available in your own environment.

1. First find the proper location to build your sweat lodge. The sweat lodge should be located close to a cool clear stream, lake, or river, or the ocean, since there must be a location to cool the body after being in the sweat lodge or sauna. If this is not possible, you can use your shower or bath to cool down after the sweat lodge.

2. Dig the pit. The pit should be in the very center of the structure and should be about two feet deep and two to three feet wide. This hole is extremely symbolic and even holy. To the Plains Indians, it traditionally represents the center of the universe.

3. Gather poles to use for the framework. Willows and other saplings work well for this purpose. Although there is no set size for a sweat lodge, gather sufficient poles to construct a lodge two to four feet high in the center and about ten feet in diameter.

4. To make the framework, plant the ends of the poles into the ground, joining the ends in the center (much like a dome in appearance). Use leather string or rope to tie the ends together. Be sure to point the entrance of the lodge to the east toward Father Sun, who has tremendous power.

5. The next step is to cover the poles with material that will keep the heat in and the light out. Rather than the animal skins that used to be used to cover sweat lodges, you may need to use heavy duty canvas sheets.

6. To use the sweat lodge, you'll need to heat rocks. The best way to do this is in an outside pit. To the Creeks, the fire used to heat the rocks represents a portion of the sun and a symbol of the Creator. The stones used in the pit represent earth as both mother and grandmother and symbolize endurance, just as the earth endures.

7. Once the rocks have been brought into the sweat lodge and placed in the pit, water should be poured onto the rocks to produce steam. The water used in the sweat lodge represents the life-giving elements of air and water.

8. An offering should be made to the fire. Native Americans often used tobacco for this purpose.

9. Drinking herbal teas in the sweat lodge can help encourage healthy skin and sweating. Herbs used for this purpose include cayenne, elderberries, ginger, pepper, peppermint, sage, and wintergreen. Drink as much tea as possible while you sweat. This will also help replenish fluids the body loses during sweating.

10. Stay in the sweat lodge for about fifteen minutes.
After the sweat, wrap up in a blanket and cool in bed for thirty to sixty minutes. Then, plunge into a nearby stream, river, or other body of water. If this isn't possible, take a cold shower or bath instead.

For more information on the spiritual aspect of healing, see the following books:

American Indian Medicine by Virgil J. Vogel (Norman: University of Oklahoma Press, 1970).

Earthway by Mary Summer Rain (New York: Pocket Books, 1990).

The Medicine Men, Oglala Sioux Ceremony and Healing by Thomas H. Lewis (Lincoln: University of Nebraska Press, 1990).

Secrets of the Sacred White Buffalo by Gary Null (Paramus, NJ: Prentice Hall, 1998).
Shamanic Healing and Ritual Drama by Åake Hultkrantz (New York: Crossroad, 1992).

Spirit Healing by Mary Dean Atwood (New York: Sterling, 1991).

Conclusion

I hope you have enjoyed reading this book as much as I've enjoyed writing it, and I hope it will accompany you in your ongoing journey to the discovery of Native American herbs and their medicinal uses.

If you found this book useful and are feeling generous, please take the time to leave a short review on Amazon so that other may enjoy this guide as well.

I leave you with good wishes and hopefully a better knowledge of the plants around us and their amazing powers. I hope you have also purchased the second and third volume of the series, so that you might explore more fully Native American herbs and herbal remedies.

• The Native American Herbalist's Bible 2 •

The Complete Field Book of the Wild Plants of North America

From Agave to Zizia. Find, Grow, and Discover the Traditional and Modern Uses of Forgotten Herbs

Linda Osceola Naranjo

Introduction

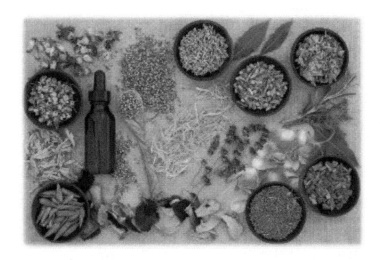

"All plants are our brothers and sisters. They talk to us and if we listen, we can hear them"
Arapaho proverb

We live in a country where the cure for virtually any disease and ailment is within our grasp. In our forests, meadows, plains, and gardens grow small, seemingly insignificant flowers and herbs, plants that we don't look twice at, and trees of which we don't even bother to learn the name. Yet, they are the key to a better, healthier, and more sustainable way of life.

Our forefathers, more attuned with nature that we could ever imagine to be, understood that and took carefully and sparingly the gifts that Nature offered to heal themselves and grow stronger. We have lost that knowledge. Only starting from the 1970s, a renewed interest in botanic medicine has uncovered the depth of the Native American knowledge of plants and their healing powers. The research has not only helped herbalists, but physicians and scientist as well that re-discovered substances that the Native Americans people knew about for hundreds of years.

You don't need to put at risk the delicate natural balance of your body by taking drugs and medications, if an easily available natural solution is just outside your door. Harvest carefully or grow your own herbs, learn to know your body and what works best for you, communicate with the nature surrounding you, and you will in a small way bring back a culture that for too long as been treated as inferior.

This book will teach how to find and treat the herbs the way the native American tribes did: from the forest to your herbalist table, but you will have to find your way to listen to your body and the plants around you.

To aid you in your holistic journey, we have decided to divide the book in three volumes. The first volume offers you a full theoretical approach to Native American medicine and the herbal medicines methods and preparations. This second volume is a complete encyclopedia of all the most relevant herbs used in traditional Native American medicine, complete with modern examples, doses, and where to find them, making it a very effective field guide. The third volume is a "recipe book" of sorts: it offers easy herbal solutions to the most common diseases a budding naturopath can encounter. It is meant as a jumping point to find your own way to treat yourself and your fellow man and will come in handy even to the most experienced herbalist.

Definitions

For each plant in the following chapter, I will enumerate the effects, or rather the medical actions of herbs and herbal medicines. The definitions for these effects are listed alphabetically for a quick reference, should the reader need it.

Alterative: herbs that gradually restore the proper function of the body and increase health and vitality, without any immediate perception of this healthful alteration. Such as stinging nettle (*urtica diocia*), yellow dock (*rumex crispus*), dandelion (*taraxacum off. radix*).

Anodyne: pain-relieving. Such as *Valeriana off.* (Valerian) and *Atropa belladonna* (Deadly Nightshade)

Anthelmintic: antiparasitic herbs or preparations that expel parasitic destroy or expel worms from the digestive system. The term is synonymous with vermifuge and antiparasitic. Such as *Artemisia absinthium* (Wormwood).

Aperient: mild laxative. Such as *Juniperus communis* (Juniper).

Aromatic: a spicy stimulant with a strong and often pleasant odour. Such as *Pimpinella anisum* (Aniseed) and *Melissa officinalis* (Lemon Balm).

Astringent: causing the tightening of skin, mucosae, and other exposed body tissues. Such as *Rubus idaeus* (Red Raspberry) and *Quercus sp* (White/Red Oak).

Antibilious: preparations that counter disorders of the liver.

Antiemetic: to stop vomiting. Such as *Chionanthus virginicus* (Fringetree)

Antileptic: anticonvulsant, soothing.

Antiperiodic: preparations preventing the recurrence of certain symptoms.

Antirheumatic: herbs or preparations used in the treatment of inflammatory arthritis, rheumatoid arthritis, and others. Such as *Sambucus nigra/canadensis* (Black Elderberry) and dandelion (*taraxacum off. radix*).

Antiscorbutic: to cure or prevent scurvy.

Antiseptic: antimicrobial herbs or preparations to reduce the possibility of infection, sepsis, or putrefaction. Such as *Hamamelis virginiana* (Witch Hazel), *Capsella bursa-pastoris* (Shepherd's Purse), and *Quercus alba* (White Oak).

Antispasmodic: to prevent or soothe spasms or craps of the muscles. Such as *Viburnum prunifolium* (Black Haw) and *Passiflora incarnata* (Passionflower).

Carminative: herbs and preparations rich in volatile oils, that increase the peristalsis of the gastric and intestinal mucosae and relieve cramping by expelling gases. Such as *Pimpinella anisum* (Anise).

Cathartic: to accelerate defecation. Such as *Juglans nigra* (Black Walnut) and *Podophyllum peltatum* (May Apple).

Cephalic: related to the treatment of headaches.

Cholagogue: to stimulate the flow of bile from the liver. Such as *Hydrastis canadensis* (Goldenseal)

Condiment: to improve the flavour of foods.

Demulcent: herbs rich in mucilage that can soothe and protect irritated or inflamed internal tissue. Such as *Althea off.* (Marshmallow leaf or root) and *Glycyrrhiza glabra* (Licorice).

Deobstruent: to clear or open the natural ducts of the fluids and secretions of the body; see aperient.

Depurative: detoxifying; see alterative.

Detergent: cleansing herbs that contain saponins. Such as *Agave Americana* (Agave).

Diaphoretic: to stimulate perspiration and the production of sweat. Such as Eupatorium perfoliatum (Boneset) and *Sambucus niger* (Elderberry).

Diuretic: to increase the secretion and flow of urine. Stimulating diuretics such as *Arctostaphylos uva-ursi* (Bearberry) and *Juniperus communis* (Juniper) either irritate the kidneys or increase the flow of blood (caffeine) to the kidneys to increase the flow of urine. Osmotic diuretics such as *Agropyron repens* (Couch Grass) and *Althea officinalis* (Marshmallow) works as unmetabolized polysaccharides change the osmotic pull of the kidneys and increase the flow of water.

Emetic: herbs that induce vomiting; first aid treatment for poisoning. Such as Lobelia (*Lobelia inflata*) and Ipecac (*Cephaelis ipecacuahana*)

Emmenagogue: to stimulate and regulate menstrual flow and function. Such as Achillea millefolium (Yarrow), Actaea racemosa (Black Cohosh), and Caulophyllum thalictroides (Blue Cohosh).

Emollient: softens and soothes the skin. Such as *Plantago major/lanceolata* (Plantain) and *Aloe barbadensis* (Aloe).

Esculent: edible.

Expectorant: herbs that help the body to remove excess mucous from the lungs, or more generally a tonic for the respiratory system. Stimulating expectorants such as *Inula helenium* (Elecampane), *Glycyrrhiza glabra* (Licorice), and *Sanguinaria canadensis* (Bloodroot) work as chemical irritants to the mucosae of the bronchiole forcing the expulsion of the congested material.

Soothing or Relaxing expectorants such as *Tussilago farfara* (Coltsfoot) and *Verbascum thapsus* (Mullein) soothe bronchial spasms and loosen mucous secretion.

Febrifuge: Abates and reduces fevers. Such as *Sambucus nigra* (Elderberry) and *Filipendula ulmaria* (Meadowsweet).

Hepatic: herbs or preparations that aid the work of the liver. Such as *Taraxacum officinalis* (Dandelion root) and *Silybum marianum* (Milk thistle).

Laxative: to promote bowel movements. Stimulating laxatives such as *Cassia angustifolia* (Senna), *Rheum palmatum* (Turkey Rhubarb), and *Rhamnus purshiana* (Cascara) contain anthraquinones which stimulate the contractions of the muscle wall of the large intestine. Osmotic laxatives such as *Althea off.* (Marshmallow) bulk up the colon by drawing water and softening the stool.

Mucilaginous: soothe and protect irritated tissues in the body. Such as *Althea off.* (Marshmallow), *Plantago lanceolata* (plantain), and *Verbascum thapsus* (Mullein).

Nervine: a remedy that has a beneficial effect on the nervous system, either relaxant, stimulant, or tonic. Such as *Hypericum perforatum* (St. John's wort), *Humulus lupulus* (Hops), and *Lavendula off.* (Lavender).

Refrigerant: cooling. Such as *Borago off.* (Borage).

Rubifacient: to increase capillary circulation and produce redness of the skin. Such as *Bryonia alba/diocia* (White Bryony).

Sedative: to reduce stress and aid sleep. Such as *Gelsemium sempervirens* (Yellow Jasmine), *Piscidia erythrina* (Jamaican Dogwood) and *Eschscholzia california* (California Poppy).

Sialogogue: to increase the secretion of saliva. Such as *Rheum palmatum* (Turkey Rhubarb).

Styptic: an astringent applied externally. See Astringent.

Tonic: herbs and preparations that are generally invigorating and strengthening.

Vermifuge: See Anthelmintic.

Native American Herbs

Agave

Century plant *(Agave americana)*, blue agave
(A. tequilana), and others

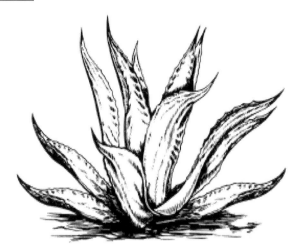

Habitat: Extreme southwestern United States—
dry areas of California, Arizona, Nevada, and
Mexico; Central and South America.

Identification: Grayish-green desert plant to
10' with long, swordlike, succulent leaves.
Produces flowers on a central fruiting spike.
Also known as American century plant,
because people came to believe that the plant
blooms only once every 100 years. This isn't
actually true: the plant does flower at a ripe
old age, blooming once in 10 to 20 years. After sending up its huge flower spear, the mother
plant will die. But the American decade plant is probably not a good name.

Taste: sweet, comparable to honey.

Medicinal Parts: The leaf and the juice.

Solvent: Water, alcohol.

Effects: anti-inflammatory, diuretic.

Traditional uses: Agave water (juice, sap) is considered anti-inflammatory and diuretic. Also
the fresh juice may raise metabolism and increase perspiration.
The sap is used for treating and sealing wounds. Cortez dropped his axe half through his thigh
and surely would have died had not the Mesoamerican natives stopped the bleeding and sealed
the wound with a compress of sticky agave leaf sap, honey, and charcoal, then bound that with
spiderwort stems.

Modern uses: Leaf waste is gathered, concentrated, and used as starter material for steroid
drugs (hecogenin). The drug Crinone, which is prescribed as a progesterone hormone
replacement therapy in certain situations around pregnancy, is produced from the Agave
sisalana species.

Agave roots contain suds-producing saponins and are used in the manufacture of soap products. In fact, if you grate agave roots, press them, and add water, you'll end up with a foaming liquid soap that can be used as shampoo, dish soap, or laundry soap.

The coarse fiber from leaves is used to make rope and fiber, such as sisal. Amazingly, sisal is strong enough to be part of the equipment used to haul elevators up and down.
Sisal is coarse and super-strong cordage, which is oiled and wrapped into the pulley systems of the elevator shaft. As the elevator cables work, they move through the pulleys, where they get lubricated by the oiled sisal fibers. This prevents friction from building up as the cables move to raise and lower the elevator in the shaft. The sap continues to be used as a demulcent and laxative.

Agave nectar is commercially processed into low glycemic index sugar or liquid sweetener, but beware! Agave sugar and nectar are high in fructose, which retards the release of insulin and actually leads to more fat formation and storage. Furthermore, evidence suggests that agave sugar or nectar may actually increase insulin resistance and fructose may increase the risk of heart disease.

Food: In the Sonoran Desert, *Agave deserti* is considered one of the best agaves for cooking. Native groups such as the Pima, Papago (Tohono O'odham), and Cahuilla Indian tribes collect and dry agave flowers, grind them into flour, and use it to make tortillas. Each plant will provide several pounds of flowers. The Papago people also ate these flower stalks as a green vegetable, while several Native American groups baked or roasted the roots and hearts of agave to make traditional cakes and breads. Navajos used baked, dried agave heads as a soup thickener.

The heart of the agave can be roasted and eaten. Baking and mashing the heart is also how the juices are extracted to ferment and distilled into tequila.

If you buy a bottle of tequila, you might see a little worm in the bottom of the bottle. This is the agave worm, also called a maguey worm or gusano. At the time of bottling, it's added as evidence of the tequila's proof; if the tequila's alcohol percentage is not high enough, the worm will rot (not very appetizing)! However, if the worm is intact and sound, the drinker can be assured that the tequila is of very good quality.

Warning: Livestock can become fatally ill from eating agave leaves — something they avoid except in cases of severe drought or when no other forage is available.
Humans have occasionally used this toxicity to their advantage: one way that indigenous people in parts of Mexico harvested fish was to put agave leaves (*A. lechuguilla*) in a stream. Any fish swimming in that area would take in the toxic water through their gills, become paralysed, and float to the water's surface, where they could be collected. This poison would not make the fish unsafe to eat (since the agave isn't toxic to humans), and any uncollected fish floating into clean water would revive and swim away.

Alder

Betulaceae *(Alnus rubra Bong.)*

Habitat: Species ranges from California to Alaska east to Idaho. Moist areas. It forms thickets along waterways. In Colorado the primary species is Alnus tenuifolia and is common in the foothills to subalpine areas.

Identification: Member of the birch family to 80' in height, often much smaller. Bark smooth and gray when young, coarse and whitish gray when mature. A. rubra bark turns red to orange when exposed to moisture. Leaves are bright green, oval, coarsely toothed and pointed. Male flowers clustered in long, hanging catkins; female seed capsule is ovoid cone. Seed nuts small, slightly winged, flat.

Medicinal Part: The bark.

Solvent: Boiling water.

Effects: Tonic, Alterative, Astringent, Cathartic.

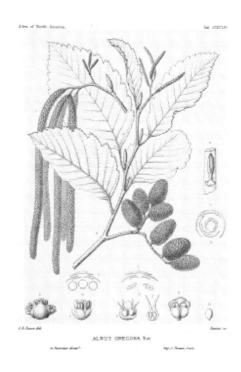

Traditional uses: Sweat-lodge floors were often covered in alder leaf, and switches of alder were used for applying water to the body and the hot rocks. Alder ashes were used as a paste with a chewing stick to clean the teeth. Cones of subspecies A. sinuata are also used for medicine, as are other alder species. Spring catkins were smashed to pulp and eaten as a cathartic (to help move the bowels). The bark was sometimes mixed with other plants in decoction and used as a tonic. Female catkins were used in decoction to treat gonorrhea. A poultice of leaves was applied to skin wounds and skin infections. In the Okanagan area of central Washington and British Columbia, First People used an infusion of new end shoots as an appetite stimulant for children. The leaf tea infusion said to be an itch- and inflammation-relieving wash for insect bites and stings and poison ivy and poison oak. Upper Tanana informants reported that a decoction of the inner bark reduces fever. An infusion of bark was used to wash sores, cuts, and wounds.

Modern uses: This is still an important warrior plant in sweat lodge ceremonies. Black alder, A. glutinosa, is endemic to the Northern Hemisphere and is used in Russia and eastern European countries as a gargle to relieve sore throat and reduce fever. Research suggests that betulin and lupeol in alder may inhibit tumor growth.

Dose and usage: The bark is high in tannin and can be used in all situations where tannin is effective such as: (internally) diarrhea, gum inflammations, and sore throats; and (externally) as a wash for cuts, hives, poison ivy, swellings and sprains. The bark tea has a shrinking, clotting, and antiseptic effect and is therefore good for wounds. The bark is best collected in the spring or fall, though is good anytime. The bark is best used fresh or of recent collection. Make a strong decoction for internal use, weak for external.

Notes: To smoke meat with alder, soak the wood chips overnight in water, then place the moist chips on coals or charcoal to smoke meat. In 1961 I saw more than a hundred Native Americans smoking fish, moose, and caribou for winter storage along a 10-mile stretch of the Denali Highway in Alaska. Hunting rules at that time required any person shooting a caribou to give some of the meat to the First People, who preserved it for winter food. Fish were flayed, stabbed through with a stick, and hung from wood weirs above a smoldering alder fire until smoked and dry. Ashes of alder were mixed with tobacco and smoked. In hardwood-poor areas of the West, alder burns slower than pine and is a suitable home-heating fuel. Bark may be stripped and soaked in water to make an orange-to-rust dye. Numerous alder species are found across North America, often in impenetrable mazes surrounding stream beds—great bear habitat, so be careful.

Food: Members of this genus provide a generous resource of firewood in the Northwest for savory barbecue cooking. The bark and wood chips are preferred over mesquite for smoking fish, especially salmon. The sweet inner bark is scraped in the early spring and eaten fresh, raw, or combined with flour to make cakes.

Aloe

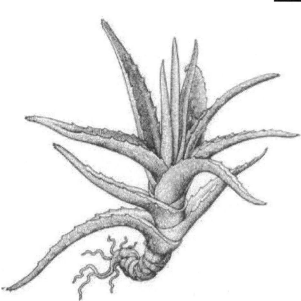

Liliacee (Aloe vera)

Habitat: Aloe, a genus of nearly 200 species of mostly South African succulent plants. The properties of this plant were known to the ancient Greeks and it has been gathered on Socotra for over 2.000 years.
Aloe thrives in warm regions and grows wild in Florida, U.S.A. It is much like succulent cactus in texture.

Identification: The leaves are usually elongated, of a deep brown or olive color, frequently pointed, blunt, or spine-toothed, sometimes blotched or mottled.
The stem is commonly short with a basal rosette of leaves.

The red or yellow tubular flowers are found on a stalk in simple or branched clusters.

These properties change somewhat in the different varieties, some species being tree—like with forked branches: for example, Aloe bainesii grows to heights of 65 ft. and is 5 ft. wide at the base.
Other species of Aloe are often cultivated in gardens of succulents, including the miniature ones grown in homes; they require strong light and careful watering.

The "American aloe" is not an Aloe, but Agave americana.

Taste: peculiar and bitter.

Powder: bright yellow.

Medicinal Parts: The insipid juice of the leaves, which is a greenish translucent salve-like substance.

Solvent: Water.

Effects: Tonic, Purgative, emmenagogue, anthelmintic.

Medicinal uses: Aloes are one of the most effective agents we have among herbal medicines, having a cleansing effect to the tissues of the stomach, liver, spleen, kidney and bladder. Does not gripe and is very healing and soothing to all the tissue, including blood and lymphatic fluids. Aloes should never be used in pregnancy, or if suffering from hemorrhoids, as it irritates the lower bowels. It's used in case of suppressed menstruation, dyspepsia, skin lesions, disease of the liver, headaches, etc.

Dose and use: In constipation, in powder form from %—2 grains, depending on age and conditions; for obstructed or suppressed menstruation, 5-10 grains twice daily; to expel thread worms dissolve the Aloe in warm water and use as an injection. The same mixture can be taken orally for several days.
Externally: powdered Aloes made into a strong decoction and rubbed over the nipples will help wean a nursing child; the association of the pleasant experience will soon find other sources due to the disagreeable bitter taste. Aloes show the same cleansing power for external application.
A piece of white linen or cotton saturated in Aloe water can be applied to fresh wounds, as well as old ones to close them quickly.
. If ulcers progress to a running stage sprinkle Aloe powder thick enough to cover the open wound and secure with clean gauze, repeating daily. The powder will absorb the morbid, fluid matter, at the same time encouraging the buildup of new, healthy tissues.
The fresh juice, or solution made from dried leaves, is soothing to tender sunburns, insect bites, over-exposure to X-ray or other emollient uses.

Warning: Do not give in cases of degeneration of the liver and gallbladder, as well as menstruation, pregnancy and hemorrhoids. As a rule, it is safe to use Aloe as it is established by Folk Medicine, but in all complicated cases the advice of medical or trained practitioners in this field should be sought.

Amaranth

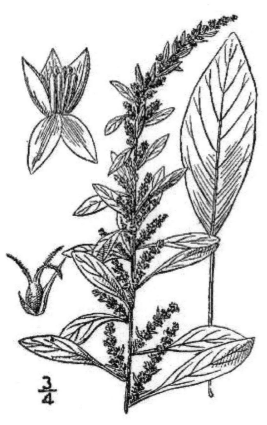

Amaranthaceae: Redroot amaranth *(Amaranthus retroflexus)*, red amaranth *(A. cruentus)*, and others

Identification: Tall, weedy-looking plant to 4' with grayish leaves, leaves alternate, flowers borne in bristly, hairy bracts in the axils of the upper leaves. Leaves diminish in size near the top of the stem as hairy flower bracts increase in size and density. Seeds are typically black, small, and numerous. Taproot and lower stem are reddish, thus the name. Leaves are ovate to rhomboid, alternate with rough margins, rough to the touch. Flowers in summer, bears edible seeds in fall.

Habitat: Numerous species growing on waste ground across the nation along the edges of prairies, margins of fields. Widely cultivated in Mexico and South America.

Medicinal Parts: Flowers and leaves. Edible seeds and shoots.

Solvent: Water.

Effects: Astringent.

Food: Native Americans have been eating amaranth seeds for thousands of years. The Apaches and Navajos used amaranth to make flour for bread, while the Aztecs and later the Tarahumara (Rarámuri) people of what is now Mexico would make pinole — toasted amaranth or cornmeal that is mixed with sugar, spices, and a bit of water and eaten as hot cereal or cooked into cakes. Amaranth flour, mixed with cornmeal, was made into dumplings, too, and the seeds were popped like popcorn.

In Mexico a traditional sweet treat called alegría (Spanish for "joy") — popped amaranth seeds mixed with honey and chocolate, sometimes with pumpkin or sunflower seeds added, too — is made in honor of the Day of the Dead and other celebrations. The recipe's origins go back as far as the Mayans and Aztecs. Amaranth has again become an important food for the descendants of those early Mayans, who grow the amaranth and make products from the seeds, including alegría, as a way to earn a livelihood and provide nutritious food for their families.

Like its cousin quinoa, amaranth is a rich source of protein and other nutrients, and it's gluten-free. One cup of uncooked seeds provides 26 grams of protein, 307 milligrams of daily calcium, 14.7 milligrams of iron requirements, and 158 micrograms of folic acid. This nutritious food is especially good for children and pregnant women, for whom it's very important to consume adequate amounts of protein, folic acid, calcium, and other essential nutrients. The folks at NASA know its value; they've recommended amaranth as one of the most nutritious foods that can be taken on space missions.

Other parts of the plant are edible, too. Young leaves are a great source of vitamin C and vitamin A, and can be eaten fresh in salads or steamed and served as a cooked vegetable. Even the roots are edible when cooked, and make a great addition to soups and casseroles.

Amaranth could become an important food in a future affected by climate change. It's easy to grow in many climates (and with limited water), adapts well to different soils, and doesn't require much fertilizer (whereas other grain crops like corn generally need good soil, abundant water, and lots of fertilizer and pesticides). And because it's so packed with nutrients, it can help reduce the rates of malnutrition wherever it's grown.
Easy to grow and packed with nutrients, amaranth will likely be an important food in a future affected by climate change.

Traditional uses: Native Americans consider this a sacred ritual plant mixed and eaten with green corn in ceremonies. Astringent leaves used to treat profuse menstruation, and the infusion was taken to treat hoarseness (Moerman, 1998). Pioneers and herbalists reported the herb as astringent and useful for treating inflammations of the mouth and throat, as well as therapy for diarrhea and ulcers.

Notes: Excellent as a pink dye

Veterinarian/Wildlife: Perfect for your bird feeder

Angelica

Apiaceae (Angelica atropurpurea L.)

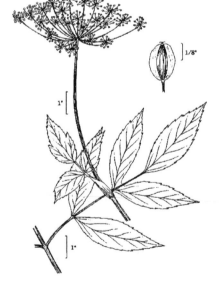

Identification: Biennial to 9'. Stem thick, erect, purple. Large compound leaves divided into three to five leaflets with hollow petioles. Upper leaves sheathed as they emerge, sheath remains around the base of the petioles. Greenish-white flowers grow in umbrellalike clusters. The root and, to a lesser degree, the seeds and leaves, have a unique and readily identifiable smell, slightly celery-like but uniquely that of angelica. After picking, if you run your fingers along the cut root, its interior has a slippery, soaplike feel. The leaves are large, divided into smaller leaflets, and a lengthened oval in shape, perhaps three to four inches long. Since angelica can be confused with water hemlock, which is quite poisonous, certain identification is a must.

Habitat: Northern tier of United States, typically east of the Mississippi River. Wet lowlands, along streams and rivers.

Medicinal Parts: Root, herb and seed.

Solvent: Boiling water.

Effects: Aromatic, Stimulant, Carminative, Diaphoretic, Expectorant, Diuretic, Emmenagogue.

Food: Whereas there is little literature on the edibility of A. atropurpurea, a similar Chinese herb, A. sinensis (dong quai), is eaten as root slices added to stir-fries or soups. A favorite eye-opener and "lip flapper" is a yin and yang cordial. To prepare it, combine 100 grams of A. sinensis root (typically available at an Asian market or drugstore) with 100 grams of whole ginseng root. Add this to ½ liter of peppermint schnapps. Saponins (phytosterols), including phytoestrogens, are drawn from the roots into the schnapps. It takes at least three weeks to get a good tincture. I use the cordial as an aperitif that balances yin and yang and boosts energy. Laplanders supposedly eat the cooked roots of A. atropurpurea.

Traditional uses: More than eighteen American Indian tribes used angelica species for medicine in a similar manner to that of Western medicinal use.
Native Americans used A. atropurpurea root decoctions to treat rheumatism, chills and fevers, and flatulence and as a gargle for sore throat. It was often used in sweat-lodge ceremonies for treating arthritis, headaches, frostbite, and hypothermia. The root was smashed and applied externally as a poultice to relieve pain.
The Creek Indians chewed the root and swallowed the juice or smoked it dry with tobacco for disorders of the stomach.
Angelica infusions were used by the Iroquois in steam baths to treat headaches and frostbite. Angelica root poultices were applied to broken bones, and angelica tea served as a topical treatment for ulcers. Angelica was also widely used as a purification herb, added to sacred pipes and burned in healing ceremonies.
A. sinensis and A. atropurpurea are used differently in Asian and Western traditions, and there are minor chemical differences between the plants too. Unless stated otherwise, assume that the uses described next are for A. sinensis, which may be purchased from herbs.com as seed or as dried roots from health-food stores and Asian markets. The root, a warming tonic, is the number-one female herb in traditional Chinese herbal medicine, and it is used to treat menstrual cramps and may improve scanty menstrual flow. As an antispasmodic it is reported helpful in reducing angina. Like other members of the Apiaceae plant family, angelica contains calcium channel blockers, similar to the drugs used to treat angina. According to Chinese practitioners, angelica improves peripheral circulation to distal parts of body.

Modern uses: German holistic healthcare professionals prescribe 3 teaspoons of dried A. sinensis infused in water to treat heartburn and indigestion. A. sinensis is used by European professionals for treating colic also. American naturopathic physicians use both species; seek out a holistic naturopathic practitioner for professional advice.

Dose and usage: Angelica is used by herbalists as a reproductive normalizer; to stimulate delayed menstruation; for cramps (reproductive or intestinal); to normalize digestion and relieve flatulence; as an expectorant during coughs and colds; as a diaphoretic and diuretic to cure urinary tract infections. It is a urinary antiseptic. It has some use in relieving joint inflammations. The part used is primarily the root, though the seeds work very well for stomach nausea. The stems and leaves have a weaker action—in Europe they are used candied as a dessert and to some extent in the liquor industry as a flavoring.
Angelica's root can be eaten in its raw, whole form, by simply carrying a portion of the root and nibbling at it from time to time. Generally, the root is used as a tincture, thirty to sixty drops up to four times a day. The seeds can be tinctured also (ten to thirty drops up to four times a day), or several seeds can be taken in raw form and chewed.

To make a tea, pour one cup of boiling water over two teaspoons of crushed angelica seeds. Let steep for thirty minutes. Strain. Take two tablespoons up to four times a day. If using angelica root, place two teaspoons of dried angelica root in a pan with three cups of water. Bring to a boil, then reduce heat and simmer until the liquid is reduced to one and a half cups. Remove from the heat and strain. Take a quarter cup up to four times daily.

Notes: Angelica roots are used as a flavoring agent for vodka, gin, cooked fish, and various jams.

Veterinarian/Wildlife: Oil from the root attracts fruit flies. Angelica is pollinated by bees, flies, and beetles. The fruit is crushed and decocted as a wash to kill head lice.

Wild Anise

Apiaceae *(Myrrhis odorata L. Scop.)*

Identification: Be careful—this is a hemlock lookalike but much smaller even when mature. Grows to less than 3'. Broken root smells like anise seed. Shiny, bright green leaves; small, white flowers in umbels. Wild anise, commonly called sweet cicely, has a sweet anise odor and taste. Flowers appear in late spring to early summer. Fruit is pyramid shaped, compressed at sides and brown to glossy black, plus or minus an 1" in length. Leaves smell like lovage and taste like anise. Short feather- or fernlike leaves are covered underneath with hairlike soft bristles, leaves deeply cleft.

Habitat: Forest dweller. Found throughout entire United States except extremes of desert, mountains. Shade preferring.

Food: Leaves and root edible, but looks like poison hemlock. Be careful. Use root to spice cooked greens and baked goods. Used as an anise substitute. Leaves can be added to salads. Cooked root can be eaten cold or pickled; try it in salads, soups.

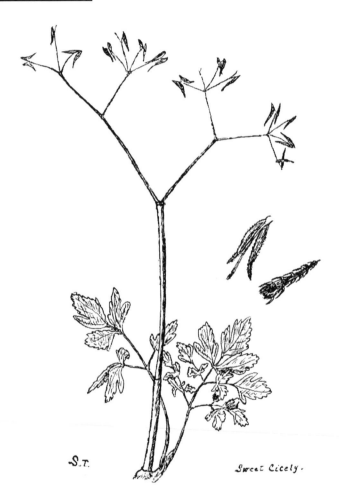

S.T.

Sweet Cicely.

Traditional uses: Used as a blood purifier and expectorant for hundreds of years. Traditionally used to treat asthma and other breathing difficulties.

Modern uses: Root tea used as an expectorant, decongestant, and digestive aid. Still considered useful in treating anemia, probably due to iron in root. As a food additive or spice, the cooked root acts as a carminative.

Dose and usage: Pick leaves for salads. Use root for food and medicine. Anethole, a volatile oil, imparts the aniselike flavor. Preparation: Root is macerated and infused in water as a tea. Keep pot or cup covered so as not to lose essential oils. Keeping macerated root in stoppered bottle of water may yield more of the aromatic, volatile oils.

Balsam Fir

Pinaceae (*Abies balsamea* L. Mill)

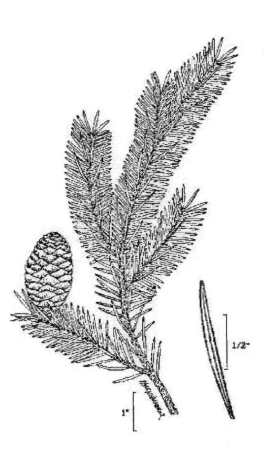

Identification: Spire-shaped evergreen to 60' in height. At higher altitudes this tree is spreading, low, more matlike. Smooth barked; bark has numerous resin pockets. Flat, stalkless needles to 1¼" in length with white stripes beneath, more thickly rounded at the base. Cones purplish to green, to 4" in length, scaly, twice as long as broad.

Habitat: Canada south through the northern tier of the eastern United States. Moist woods and their fringes.

Medicinal parts: Resin, root, needles, and bark

Effects: Analgesic, antiseptic

Food: The needle infusion is a relaxing tea, traditionally considered a laxative.

Traditional uses: Native Americans used the resin to treat burns and wounds and to soothe sores, scrapes, insect bites, stings, and bruises. Tea from needles was used to treat upper respiratory problems: asthma, bronchitis, and colds. Leaves were stuffed into pillows as a general cure-all. Children chewed raw sap to treat colds and sore throats. In sweat lodges, balsam gum was applied to hot, wet stones and the smoke inhaled as a cure for headaches. Branches were steamed to treat arthritis (rheumatism). A bark decoction will induce sweating as a way of treating acute infections.

Many tribes, including the Algonquin, Woodlands Cree, Iroquois, Menominee, Micmac, Ojibwa, and Potawatomi treat colds with a tea made from the sap or bark. The Ojibwa also inhale the smoke from the needlelike leaves to treat colds.

The gum of the fir makes an effective treatment and also a protective coating for burns, wounds, and cuts. The Chippewa inhale steam created by melting balsam gum to relieve headaches, while the Iroquois have used the steam created from a decoction of the branches to relieve rheumatism and as an aid to childbirth.

Modern uses: The resin obtained from bark blisters is considered antiseptic and is an integral ingredient in many salves and lotions, including ointments and creams used to treat hemorrhoids. Proprietary mixtures incorporating balsam resin are sold to treat diarrhea and coughs.

Dose and usage: To make a tea, cover one teaspoon of the bark with two cups of water in a pan and bring to a boil. Boil for thirty minutes and strain. Take a quarter cup a day.

Balsam Root

Asteraceae (*Balsamorhiza sagittata* [Pursh] Nutt.)

Identification: There are numerous species. B. sagittata grows 1' to 2' in height and is found in clumps. Leaves basal, petioled, and arrow shaped; hairy, rough to the touch; from 8" to 12" in length. Flowers yellow, long stalked. Up to twenty-two yellow rays encircle the yellow disc of florets.

Habitat: Foothills and higher elevation of the Rockies from Colorado north to Canada and west to British Columbia. Dry or well-drained sunny slopes. This plant is widespread in the Bitterroots and other Idaho wilderness areas and on the south-facing slopes of Rainbow Lake, Absaroka/Beartooth Wilderness.

Medicinal parts: The whole plant.

Effects: Antiseptic, antibacterial

Balsamorhiza macrolepis   Balsamorhiza sagittata   Balsamorhiza serrata

© Regents of the University of California

Food: Young leaves and shoots are edible, as well as young flower stalks and young stems. They may be steamed or eaten raw. Peeled roots are also eaten but are bitter unless cooked slowly to break down the indigestible polysaccharide (inulin). The roots may be cooked and dried, then reconstituted in simmering water before eating. Seeds are eaten out of hand or pounded into a meal used as flour. The roasted seeds can be ground into pinole. The Nez Perce roasted and ground the seeds, which they then formed into little balls by adding grease.

Traditional uses: Native Americans used the wet leaves as a wound dressing and a poultice over burns. The sticky sap sealed wounds and was considered antiseptic. Although balsam root is bitter when peeled and chewed, it contains inulin that may stimulate the immune system, providing protection from acute sickness such as colds and flu. The sap is considered antibacterial and antifungal. A decoction of the leaves, stems, and roots was taken for stomachache and colds. The root was also used for treating gonorrhea and syphilis. In the sweat lodge, balsam root smoke and steam is reported to relieve headaches. It is considered a warrior plant, and in smudging ceremonies it is a disinfectant and inhaled for body aches. The chewed root was used as a poultice over sores, wounds, and burns.

Barberry

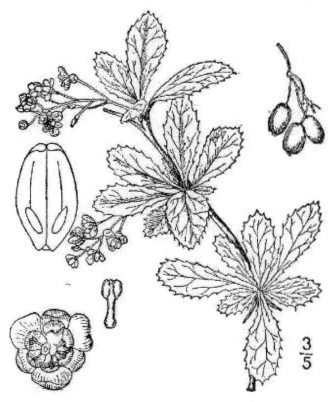

Berberidaceae (*Berberis canadensis* P. Mill.)

Identification: Thorny shrub, thorns to 1" in length. Grows to 7' tall, branches grooved, with tear drop–shaped, succulent leaves, alternate in whorled clusters; fruit round to ovate, scarlet color when ripe, tart tasting (sour). Flowers are yellow with six sepals hanging in clusters.

Habitat: Found in open woodland (dry) and edges of woods, northern tier of states from coast to coast; however, most prevalent east of the plains.

Medicinal parts: Berries, bark, and leaves

Solvents: Alcohol, water.

Effects: Tonic, purgative, antiseptic

Food: Berries cooked and juiced, dried and powdered for mush. Fruit when ripe may be cooked to make jelly. Juice: Cook fruit and extract juice with a sieve, pantyhose, or cheesecloth, and dilute and sweeten to taste. Berries may be dried, then pounded to powder or paste and cooked like hot cereal.

Traditional uses: Native Americans made good use of the barberry bush. The berries were eaten raw or made into jam, the root was used raw or boiled as a flavoring and in stew, and the wood and the bark make a yellow dye.
Cherokee remedy was to scrape free bark, place in a gourd with water, drop a hot stone in water, then drink the resultant tea for diarrhea. Micmac, Mohegan, and other tribes used pounded bark on mouth sores, sore gums, or sore throat. Placed in mouth, pounded roots induce salivation and promote healing. Mohegan used decoction of berries for reducing fevers. Shinnecock used the bitter leaves in decoction as a liver tonic.

Modern uses: Barberry contains an alkaloid called berberine, which has demonstrated significant antimicrobial activity against bacteria, fungi, protozoans, and viruses. A root decoction makes an effective topical wash for cuts and bruises.

The root bark is a source of vitamin C. Root bark for mouth sores and sore throat, like other Berberis and Mahonia spp. Decocted leaves used as a liver tonic. Increases bile flow in laboratory animals and stimulates peristalsis. Homeopathic and allopathic uses to treat liver disease (Thomson, 2007, p. 66). Root bark in decoction or infusion used as a diuretic for urinary tract infections, gout, diarrhea, arthritis.

Dose and use: To prepare tea from the berries, pour one cup of boiling water over one to two teaspoons of the ripe berries (either whole or crushed). Let steep for fifteen minutes and then strain. If using barberry roots, place half a teaspoon of the dried and powdered root bark in a pan with one cup of water. Bring to a boil and boil for twenty to thirty minutes. Remove from the heat, cool, and strain. You may want to sweeten with honey. Drink up to one cup per day of the tea, one tablespoon at a time.

Fruit can also be used as a wine or alcohol tincture for treating infections and colds.

Warning: An overdose of the root bark can cause diarrhea, kidney irritation, light stupor, nosebleeds, and vomiting.

Notes: You can use the berries to make a grayish-brown dye. Native Americans used an application of crushed berries to waterproof baskets.

Veterinarian/Wildlife: Several herbal formulas for horses incorporate uva-ursi, including formulas for joint-rebuilding/protecting supplements, training mixes, and fertility boosters.

Bearberry

Ericaceae *(Arctostaphylos uva-ursi L. Spreng)*

Identification: Trailing shrub, low lying, prostrate and mat forming. Leaves dark, evergreen, leathery, smooth edged, obovate or spatula shaped, less than ¾" wide. Alpine variety of bearberry has larger leaves. Fruit is a dry red berry. Also known as kinnikinnick or uva-ursi.

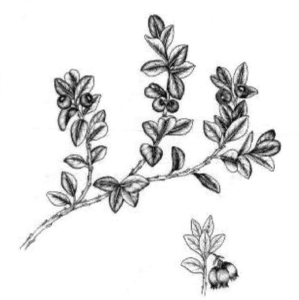

Habitat: Northern United States from East to West, and Canada in boggy and relatively dry areas, at the base of pines, tamarack, and juniper.

Medicinal parts: The leaves.

Solvents: Alcohol, water.

Effects: Astringent, Diuretic, Tonic.

Food: The berries are dry and mealy and lack flavor, so they were traditionally cooked with animal fat or mixed with fish eggs (such as salmon eggs) and stronger-tasting foods. Berries may be dried and then smashed into a flourlike meal. First People of the Northwest used this flour like a spice with meat and organ meats. People of the Bella Coola Nation mixed berries in fat and ate them; Lower Chinook peoples dried the berries and then mixed them with fat for food. Many Native Americans boiled the berries with roots and vegetables to make a soup. You can sauté the berries in grease until crisp, then place them in cheesecloth or pantyhose and pound them to a mash. Add the mash to cooked fish eggs and stir, pound in some more mash and eggs, mix, then sweeten to taste. Berries are an aromatic and flavor-enhancing addition to wild fowl and game.

Traditional uses: The whole plant was infused in water and mixed with grease from a goose, duck, bear, or mountain goat. Then glue cooked from an animal's hoof, either horse or deer, was mixed into the grease. The resulting salve was used on sores, babies' scalps, and rashes. An infusion of aerial parts was gargled as a mouthwash to treat canker sores and sore gums. Dried leaves and stems were ground and used as a poultice over wounds. An infusion of leaves, berries, and stems was taken orally for cleaning kidneys and bladder complaints as a diuretic. The same beverage had an analgesic effect on back pain and sprains. Berries were eaten or infused with whole plant for colds. Kwakiutl peoples smoked the leaves for the reported narcotic effect. Dried leaves were crushed to a powder and sprinkled on sores. Leaves and tobacco were mixed and placed in religious bundles for spiritual healing. Pioneers used the leaf infusion as a diuretic, astringent, and tonic (Moerman, p. 87).

Modern uses: Commission E–approved to treat infections of the urinary tract. It is commercially available dried, powdered in capsules, and as whole leaves for tea. There are numerous homeopathic preparations. The hot tea is considered styptic, astringent, and antibacterial. The tea as a diuretic increases urine flow. Also the tea internally and externally is considered antimicrobial and anti-inflammatory, and it has prevented kidney stone formation in lab animals.

Dose and use: Can be taken orally as follows: soak the leaves in sufficient alcohol or brandy to cover, for one week or more. Place 1 teaspoonful of the soaked leaves in 1 cup of boiling, or cold, water, drink 2-3 cups a day. Quantity of the tincture to be given in the same manner, 10-25 drops in water three or more times a day, according to symptoms. The tea can be made without the brandy or alcohol, if desired, preparing as you would ordinary tea. Effective if mixed with tincture of Quaking aspen (Populus tremuloides) 2-15 drops, tincture of Bearberry (Arctostaphylos) 10-20 drops.

Warning: Do not use during pregnancy or while nursing. Avoid eating acidic foods when using the tea to treat urogenital and biliary tract diseases. Prolonged use of uva-ursi may damage the liver and inflame and irritate the bladder and kidneys. Its use is not recommended for children, and it should not be used if you have high blood pressure.

Notes: You can use the berries to make a grayish-brown dye. Native Americans used an application of crushed berries to waterproof baskets.

Veterinarian/Wildlife: Several herbal formulas for horses incorporate uva-ursi, including formulas for joint-rebuilding/protecting supplements, training mixes, and fertility boosters.

Black Cohosh

Ranuculaceae *(Actaea racemosa L. Nutt.)*

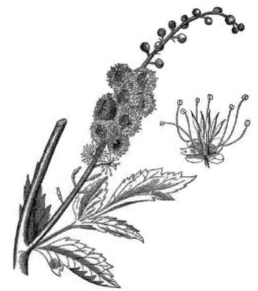

Identification: Perennial to 5½' in height. Rhizome blackish, knotty, tough. Leaves double pinnate, smooth, serrated. Flower raceme drooping, with three to eight petals. Sepals enclose flower bud.

Habitat: Northern United States and southern Canada. Primarily east of the plains in forests.

Medicinal Part: The root.

Solvent: Boiling water enhances the properties of the root but dissolves only partially; alcohol dissolves wholly.

Effects: Alterative, Diuretic, Diaphoretic, Expectorant, Anti- spasmodic, Sedative (arterial and nervous), Cardiac stimulant (safer than Digitalis), Emmenagogue.

Traditional uses: The root (rhizome) is the medicinal part. Root infusions were used to induce abortions, stimulate menstruation, and promote lactation. An alcohol infusion of the root was used to treat rheumatism. The infused root was taken to treat coughs and was said to be cathartic and stimulating, a tonic and blood purifier. Pulverized roots in hot bathwater were used as a soak to alleviate arthritis pain.

Modern uses: The plant extract is Commission E–approved for premenstrual syndrome and menopausal complaints. Commercial preparations are used to treat female conditions including uterine spasms (cramps), menstrual pain, hot flashes, mild depression, vaginal atrophy, and menopause. The estrogenic effect reduces luteinizing hormone levels. A recent study of the use of Remifemin, a proprietary black cohosh extraction, significantly reduced hot flashes and psyche disturbances in a trial group of 304 postmenopausal women (Friede, Liske, et al., Obstetric Gynecology 105 [2005]: 1074–83). The study results confirmed the efficacy and tolerability of an isopropanolic extract of black cohosh. Forty-six percent of breast cancer survivors who received a black cohosh preparation were free of hot flashes, sweating, and other symptoms of anxiety and sleep disturbances related to premenopausal breast-cancer treatment (Jacobson, Journal of Clinical Oncology 19, no. 10 [2001]: 2739–45). And a 2003 study showed an increase of bone formation in postmenopausal women (Wuttke et al., Maturitas 44 [2003]: S67–S77). Holistic health practitioners still use the plant for treating fever, arthritis, and insomnia.

Dose and use: The tincture should be made from the fresh root, or that which has recently been dried; 2 oz. to 1 pint of alcohol (96 per cent proof) taken 5-15 drops four times a day. As a tea 1 teaspoonful of the cut root to 1 cup of boiling water three times a day, or 15—30 drops of the tincture added to 1 cup of water, sweetened with honey. Externally: The bruised root was used by the Indians as an antidote for snake bites, which was applied to the wound, and the juice, in very small amounts, was taken orally.

Warning: Consult a licensed holistic health-care practitioner before using this herb for dysmenorrhea, hormone replacement therapy, or menopausal symptoms. Avoid completely if you are lactating or pregnant.

Notes: The United Kingdom health-care products regulatory agency (MHRA) and the European Medicines Agency (EMEA) have warned patients to stop using black cohosh if they develop signs suggestive of liver toxicity (blood in urine, tiredness, loss of appetite, yellowing of skin or eyes, stomach pain, nausea, vomiting, or dark urine). In the United Kingdom a warning must appear on the label of black cohosh products. For details visit herbalgram.org and search "black cohosh regulations."

Veterinarian/Wildlife: Black cohosh is used in a proprietary horse product called Fertility Boost.

Black Haw

Viburnum prunifolium, (N.O.: Caprifoliaceae)

Habitat: Black haw is found in most of the North American states, more abundantly from New York to Florida.

Identification: It's an erect bushy shrub or tree from 10-25 ft. tall, 10 in. of trunk diameter. The bark is irregular, transversely curved and greyish brown, or where the outer bark has scaled off brownish-red; inner surface reddish brown. The root bark is cinnamon in color and tastes bitter and astringent. The deep-green leaves are broadly elliptical or obovate, finely and sharply toothed, the under-surface smooth, 1-3 in. long. The flowers bloom from May to June in small white clusters 2-4 in. across and 3-5 lobes in each flower. The fruit known as Black haw is edible, but to some unbearably sweet. They are shiny black; cadet blue on red stems.

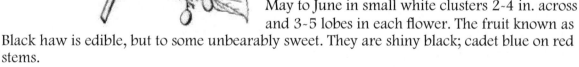

Medicinal parts: Root bark (preferred), bark of stems and branches.

Solvents: Water, alcohol.

Effects: Diuretic, Tonic, Antispasmodic, Nervine, Astringent.

Uses: To expectant mothers under risk of abortion, Black haw is an almost infallible remedy. The preparation for this purpose should be anticipated two or three weeks before the expected reoccurrence of the misfortune and continued for about two weeks after any disturbance. If there are no more symptoms during the last weeks, discontinue until after delivery.

A decoction of this plant will generally alleviate chills and fever and usually gives speedy relief in palpitation of the heart and is a valuable agent in diarrhea and dysentery. Notice that the herbs that have healing qualities on the stomach and intestinal tract are also effective for symptoms in the mouth and throat.

Dose: 1 oz. to 1 pint of boiling water taken in tablespoonful amounts three or four times a day; 1 teaspoonful of the tincture, three or four times a day. As a tea and decoction it is used for painful menstruation, excessive menstrual bleeding, cramps and hysteria. Sometimes associated with and used as a heart tonic, to improve blood circulation, kidney and bladder. Bark decoction for cramps. Berries for ulcers. Leaves as tea and decoction.

Bloodroot

Papavaraceae *(Sanguinaria canadensis L.)*

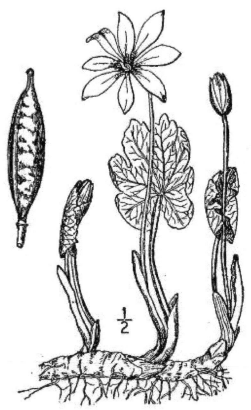

Habitat: Eastern forests south to Florida, west to Minnesota, and north to Manitoba. Damp, rich forests, along forest trails.

Identification: Perennial to 7" in height. Rhizome thick and slightly curved; exudes red liquid when cut; rootlets are reddish. Leaves down covered, grayish green, and clasping; growing in a basal rosette, with five to nine lobes, accented underneath with protruding ribs. Flower is solitary with eight to twelve white petals. This is a short-lived, early spring bloomer. Also known as red puccoon or red Indian paint.

Medicinal parts: The root

Solvents: Water, alcohol.

Effects: Expectorant, antimicrobial, anasethetic

Uses: The extract from this toxic plant is antispasmodic and warming. Native Americans discovered that the herb induced vomiting. Pioneers and First People used the root extraction in cough medicines and to treat rheumatism, fevers, and laryngitis. Some folk practitioners suggest that a very small dose works as an appetite stimulant. This may be attributed to the bitter alkaloids that stimulate the digestive system reflexively. The root juice was reportedly used to treat warts. It is anesthetic. Other reported uses were for treating bronchitis, throat infections, asthma, and other lung ailments.

Research shows that sanguinarine and chelerythrine found in bloodroot have anticancer properties. Cancer of nose and ear has responded to topical applications of bloodroot extract in research trials. It is still used topically as an anti-inflammatory. Sanguinarine, although toxic, has low oral toxicity and is antiseptic. Small amounts of it are used in a name-brand mouthwash and toothpaste.

There are reports that the red bloodroot exudate, when thinned with water and applied to the skin, was an effective mosquito repellent. Perhaps the red skin of Native Americans observed by the invading Europeans was actually bloodroot applied as a mosquito repellent. The effect of long-term exposure of sanguinarine to the skin is unknown.

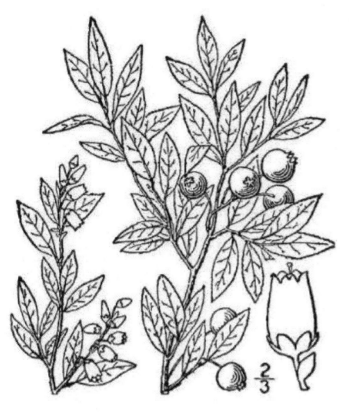

Blueberry

Ericaceae *(Vaccinium spp.)*

Habitat: Northern tier states from coast to coast. Wetlands, lowlands, and highlands, including eastern and western mountains. One of the principle species is V. myrtillus, known simply as Bilberry, which is found in acid soil, in forests, heaths, rocky barrens, bog and tundra.

Identification: Deciduous shrub from 1' to 15' tall. Sharp-edged green branches. Leaves alternate, ovate and oblong, finely serrated. Flowers greenish tinged with pink, ¼" long, containing eight to ten stamens shorter than the styles. Globular fruit blue black, often frosted, with numerous seeds dispersed through the purple pulp. There are numerous species that vary significantly. The terms "blueberry" and "bilberry" may be used interchangeably.

Medicinal parts: Leaves and berries.

Solvents: alcohol and boiling water.

Effects: Diuretic, Refrigerant, Astringent.

Food: This highly nutritious fruit may be eaten fresh, dried, stewed, or as a jam or marmalade. Leaves can be made into tea.

We have energy bars; the Iroquois, and other Native American tribes, had pemmican. This high-energy food was a mixture of meat (often buffalo or fish), nuts and seeds, animal fat, and berries or other types of fruit. They called these pemmican cakes, and they were a way to preserve food for winter and provide portable nutrition for hunting and other trips. Blueberries and other fruits were first dried like raisins, then added to the cakes. Our modern high-energy trail bars are really just a version of those early pemmican cakes — minus the meat and animal fat — usually with oats or other grains added.

Traditional uses: Native Americans used a decoction of fresh or dried berries to treat diarrhea. The Iroquois used a whole aerial part decoction as a topical application to dermatitis. Bog blueberry (V. uliginosum) leaves were infused in water and sugar and taken as a tonic by women after childbirth. Blueberries are a good source of vitamin C and have a folk use to prevent scurvy. Dried pulverized leaves were infused and taken for nausea. Other Native American uses may be found in Moerman's Native American Ethnobotany (Moerman, 1998). Pioneers used the leaves in decoction for treating diabetes. Berry tea was taken to treat mouth sores and inflammations.

Modern uses: The use of fresh and dried fruits and dried leaves is Commission E–approved for treating diarrhea and inflammation of the pharynx and mouth. The fruit is considered an antioxidant and a capillary protectant that may improve blood flow to the feet, brain, hands, eyes, and other distal areas. It is antiatherosclerotic, antiplatelet aggregating, antiglaucoma, and may provide protection from night blindness. Research suggests it may prevent varicose veins. Blueberry has induced the release of dopamine. And it may be helpful as adjunct nutritional support for Alzheimer's disease.

The rich purple-blue color of blueberries is a sign of their high levels of anthocyanins: powerful antioxidants that are important for vascular health, especially in the eyes. Medical research has shown that the anthocyanins found in blueberries and in their European cousins, bilberries, are good allies in the treatment of macular degeneration. During World War II, bomber pilots ate blueberries, because they believed that the fruit would improve their night vision. (Although some modern research has confirmed this benefit, other studies suggest that while blueberries help reduce eyestrain and improve weak eyesight, the fruit may not actually affect night vision in healthy individuals.)

Dose and usage: Place two or three handfuls of Bilberry in a bottle and pour a good, real brandy over them. Secure with a good fitting cap or cork. The longer the tincture stays the more powerful a medicine will this berry spirit be. Violent, continuous diarrhea accompanied by pain, is stopped by taking 1 tablespoonful of Bilberry brandy in 1/4 pint of water; repeat every 8 or 10 hr. For diarrhoea, dysentery and similar complaints, a decoction of the leaves will bring relief.

Of the leaves, 1 teaspoonful to 1 cup of boiling water. In the Herbalist by J. E. Meyers: "A mixture of equal parts of Bilberry leaves, Thyme, and Strawberry leaves makes an excellent tea."

Eat a fistful of blueberries daily when experiencing extended periods of bowel discomfort, gas, or diarrhea. Dry the berries in a food dryer and store them in the freezer to treat winter stomach problems—a good all-around tonic.

Boneset

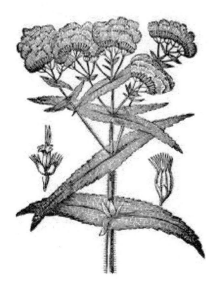

Asteraceae (*Eupatorium perfoliatum* L.)

Identification: Perennial to 5' in height. Plant rises from hairy, horizontal root-stock. Stems and leaves hairy, rough. Leaves opposite, to 7" in length, lance shaped, tapering to a point, fused around the stem at the base. The stem appears to grow through the fused leaf. White flowers are florets that form large convex head at the top of the plant. Fruit is tufted.

Habitat: Eastern United States. Thickets and wetlands, open wet prairies, marshes.

Medicinal parts: Leaves and whole aerial parts.

Solvents: alcohol and water.

Effects: Febrifuge, diaphoretic, tonic, laxative.

Traditional uses: The leaf tea was considered an excellent nineteenth-century remedy to break fevers associated with acute infections. The leaf tea was considered immune stimulating and used to treat colds, influenza, malaria, arthritis, painful joints, pneumonia, and gout and to induce sweating. Whole aerial parts of plant were applied as a poultice torelieve edema, swellings, and tumors.
This Native American cure-all was poulticed over bone breaks to help set bones. Taken internally the infusion of the aerial parts was cathartic and emetic. The infusion was also used as a gargle to treat sore throat. Other uses included treating hemorrhoids, stomach pain, and headache; reducing chills; and alleviating urinary problems.

Modern uses: Homeopaths use a microdose to treat colds, flu, and other febrile conditions. The dried and commuted aerial parts of the herb when infused in water are reported to be immunostimulating and are taken to fight colds, infections, flu, and other acute infections. More research is necessary.

Dose and usage: Infusion: 1-2 tsp herb/cup water; during fevers 1 cup every half hour as hot as possible.

Warning: Small doses (but larger than homeopathic prescriptions) of the herb are laxative and diuretic, whereas larger doses may induce catharsis and vomiting. Pyrrolizidine alkaloids present in this plant make it potentially dangerous to consume in any form, as these alkaloids have a liver-destroying capacity. Never use boneset without the consultation of a licensed holistic health-care practitioner.

California Poppy

Papaveraceae *(Eschscholzia californica* Cham.*)*

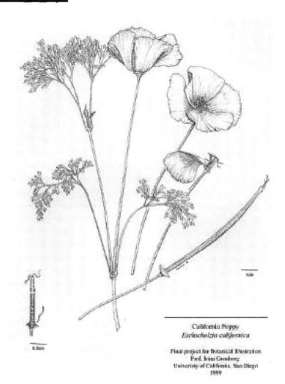

California Poppy
Eschscholzia californica

Final project for Botanical Illustration
Prof. Irina Gronborg
University of California, San Diego
1989

Identification: Annual or perennial, 15" to 40" tall. Leaves few, bluish green, tapering to a point, feathery or fernlike. Brilliant yellow-orange solitary flowers to 2" wide. Cup- or bowl-shaped seed receptacle contains several chambers filled with tiny seeds. Hundreds of species.

Habitat: California to British Columbia. Open areas, roadsides, dry clearings. Also in gardens nationwide.

Traditional uses: Aerial parts are harvested, dried, and infused as a sleep-inducing sedative. It has been used for anxiety, for nervousness, and as an antispasmolytic. It is considered a warming agent and a diuretic and has an analgesic effect. Folk use includes treating nocturnal urinating in children. Native Americans used the milky sap of the leaves as an analgesic to relieve toothaches. Leaves were also placed under children at bedtime to induce sleep. The white resin from seedpods was rubbed on a nursing mother's breast to promote lactation.

Members of the Costanoan tribe prepared the flowers as a strong tea to rinse their hair, to kill head lice. The Ohlone people crushed the seeds and mixed them with bear fat as a hair tonic dressing. Tribes in the Mendocino area juiced the roots to treat many different ailments, from headaches to stomachaches to toothaches, and nursing mothers would wash their breasts with the root juice to help dry the flow of milk when it was time to wean their babies; Pomo women made a poultice or a strong tea from the mashed seedpods and applied it to their breasts for the same purpose.

However, several tribes believed the plant to be poisonous and avoided its use.

The Yaqui Indians scattered the flowers of California poppy (E. mexicana, which they called hoohi e'es) ahead of processions during special ceremonial events, a tradition later adopted by the Gileño and Pima tribes of the Southwest, who would scatter the flowers at Easter time just outside the church entrance and ahead of processional walks.

Women from the Cahuilla Indian tribe applied the pollen as eye shadow, and as body paint for special occasions.

Modern uses: Californidine, an alkaloid in the plant, is used as a sleep aid and sedative by a few qualified holistic medicine practitioners. These qualities have been proven in animal studies only. Homeopathic preparations are used to treat insomnia and used under professional supervision.

Warning: Not to be used during pregnancy.

Notes: This attractive, deep-rooted, spreading plant is a colorful addition to your garden and provides edible seeds for baked goods. In California it is illegal to pick this plant, as it is the state flower. In addition to being a key provider for wildlife, California poppy is frequently included in wildflower seed mixes used for restoration and roadside plantings in California, where the poppies are helpful in managing soil erosion.

Cascara Sagrada (Buckthorn)

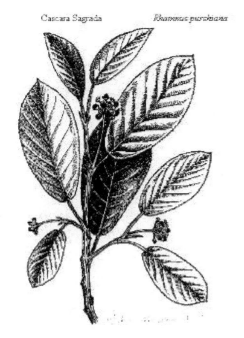

Cascara Sagrada   Rhamnus purshiana

Rhamnaceae (*Rhamnus cathartica* L.; *R. purshiana* [DC.] Cooper)

Identification: Bush or small tree 4' to 20' tall. Many branched, thornless, densely foliated. When mature, the bark is gray brown with gray-white lenticels. Leaves thin, hairy on the ribs, fully margined, elliptical to ovate, 2" in length. Greenish-white flowers are numerous and grow on axillary cymes. Flowers are very small, and five petals. The ripe fruit is red to black purple with two or three seeds. *R. purshiana* (cascara buckthorn) is taller, to 30", with leaves that have twenty to twenty-four veins. White flowers are in clusters.

Habitat: *R. cathartica* found in the dunelands of Lake Michigan and other lake dune areas. *R. purshiana*: foothills of British Columbia, Idaho, Washington, Montana, and Oregon.

Solvents: Diluted alcohol, boiling water.

Medicinal Part: The bark and root.

Effects: Laxative

Traditional uses: Prior to World War II, you could find cascara tablets over the counter as a laxative in lieu of Ex-Lax or the like. Native Americans used the bark infusion as a purgative, laxative, and worm-killing tea. An infusion of the twigs and fruit in decoction was used as an emetic. Curing the bark for a year is said to reduce its harshness.

Modern uses: The bark extract of R. purshiana is a powerful laxative. It is Commission E–approved for treating constipation. The laxative response may last eight hours.

Warning: The drug should never be used to clear intestinal obstructions. Bark infusion is considered a cleansing tonic, but chronic, continuous use may be carcinogenic. Use only under the care of a physician, holistic or otherwise. The berries are not edible.

Dose and usage: The bark should be collected in the spring and early summer when it is easily peeled from the wood. The bark should then be stored for at least one year (up to 3) in order to allow for its most bitter components to decompose: dry in the shade.

Cascara is indicated for chronic constipation. It's a gentle, tonifying laxative that can be take in the form of powdered bark, decoction of root, or tincture.

Catnip

Lamiaceae *(Nepeta cataria L.)*

Identification: A perennial that grows to 3.5'. Erect and many branched stems. Leaves are grayish green, giving the plant a whitish gray appearance. Leaves 1" to 3", are ovate and serrated with a gray underside. Leaf petiole to 1.5" long. Flower spike has a large cluster of individual flowers attached with short pedicles.

Habitat: Across North America, border to border, coast to coast: In gardens, along roadsides, and over waste ground. Tolerates well-drained, dry areas.

Solvents: Diluted alcohol, boiling water.

Medicinal Part: The Whole herb.

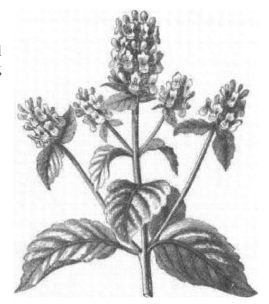

Effects: Carminative, Stimulant, Tonic, Diaphoretic, Emmenagogue, Antispasmodic

Traditional uses: Aerial parts (primarily leaves) of the plant in infusion are a bitter, astringent, and cooling antispasmodic. Catnip leaf and flower teas provide a mild sedative effect. It is antiflatulent and may settle a colicky baby (check with your holistic health-care professional before using it in this manner). Also used to soothe the digestive tract. May provide relief from menstrual cramps by mildly stimulating menstruation. The herbal tea promotes sweating, thereby lowering fever in acute infections, and like many herbal teas it is a mild diuretic.

Modern uses: Naturopaths use it to treat colic and upset stomach in children (Chevallier, 1996). Catnip may be tinctured and used as a rub for rheumatic and arthritic joints. The tea is also used to stimulate the gallbladder, and is a cleansing herb for the urinary system. Combinations: Naturopaths combine catnip leaves with elderflowers for treating acute infections. Another combination as a sleep aid is catnip, valerian root, and hops. This combination is also used to reduce stress and as a relaxant.

Warning: Not to be used during pregnancy.

Notes: Start catnip indoors and transplant it when it is at least a foot tall. Maybe then it will survive the onslaught of drug-seeking felines. Actinidine, an iridoid glycoside, is the cat-stimulating chemical of the plant. This is one of my favorite teas and should be prepared from the fresh herb in a cold infusion as its physiologically active constituents are volatile and reduced by drying. Typical dosage is three cups per day.

Veterinarian/Wildlife: Cats' drug of choice: feline stimulant and intoxicant, but a human calming agent.

Cattail

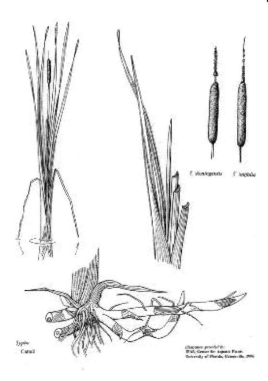

Typhaceae *(Typha latifolia L.; T. angustifolia L.)*.

Identification: Distinctive perennial to 8' tall, lance-shaped wild grass of the marsh. Two hot-dog-like flower heads in the spring: upper flower head is male, lower head female. After pollinating, the upper head disperses and disappears. Cattails grow in large stands and colonize handsomely. Two species are the broad-leafed cattail (Typha latifolia) and narrow-leafed cattail (Typha angustifolia).

Habitat: Nationwide on wet ground, edges of lakes, slow streams, marshes, shallow ponds, any wet and rich ground.

Dose and usage: Cattail roots are polysaccharide rich. Beat the roots into water and use the starchy water as a wash over sunburn. The ashes of burned cattail leaves are styptic and antimicrobial; use them to dress and seal wounds. Ash from burned leaves helps seal and keep wounds clean.

Traditional uses: Indigenous North Americans have been weaving with cattail leaves for more than 12,000 years; the leaves thatched roofs and were woven into mats and baskets. Early settlers used cattail stems and leaves to weave rush seats for their chairs.
Cattails have also been a food plant since at least 800 CE; there are caves in Ohio where archaeologists found preserved evidence of cattails eaten in meals. The Blackfoot and the Northern Paiute tribes and early colonists roasted the seeds and dried the roots, then ground them into flour to make cakes, mush porridge, and bread. Other indigenous groups, like the Yuma, mixed the pollen with water and kneaded it into little cakes, which they baked. The juicy hearts of young spring shoots were eaten as a cooked vegetable, and immature green flower heads were boiled and eaten similarly to how we eat corn on the cob (it even tastes similar!)

Notes: Cattail pollen is very flammable and has a tendency to burst when ignited; in fact, it's been part of some formulas for making fireworks for at least 200 years. In the mid-1800s, miners and settlers found that they could wire the mature brown flower heads of cattail to sticks, dip them in oil or beeswax, and use them as slow-burning torches. This practice was later replaced with safer alternatives like miners' canvas caps that had a candle or lamp bracket, eliminating the need to use cattail torches. Today enthusiasts of primitive survival skills mix cattail fluff with oil or beeswax to shape a rustic, but useful, type of candle lighting.

Chamomile

Asteraceae *(Matricaria matricarioides; Chamomilla recutita L.; Chamaemelum nobile L.)*

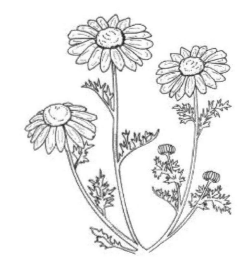

Identification: Unlike the domestic herb cultivated chamomile, wild chamomile or pineapple weed has a small yellow flower, ½" wide—without the white rays (petals) of chamomile. It is somewhat prostrate and spreading, many branched with severely cut leaves; rayless flowers are conspicuous and pineapple scented, unmistakable.

Habitat: Widespread, along roadsides, pathways, waste ground, low and high impacted soils, throughout the country east to west especially along paths and roads in the Northwest and mountainous areas.

Medicinal parts: Flowers and herb.

Solvents: Water, alcohol.

Effects: Stomachic, Antispasmodic, Tonic stimulant (volatile oil), Carminative, Diaphoretic, Nervine, Emmenagogue, Sedative.

Food: Tea, fresh flowers preferred over dried. Fresh pineapple weed is more powerful than chamomile. Leaves edible but bitter. Native Americans pulverized the dried plant and mixed it with meat and berries as a preservative.

Traditional uses: Pineapple weed is used just like chamomile. Pioneers drank the fresh flower tea as an antispasmodic carminative to aid digestion, prevent ulcers, and relieve arthritis pain. Said to soothe the nerves. Warm tea may relieve toothache pain. Native Americans used the herb in the same way, primarily for relieving stomach pain. It is considered a female plant, applied wet to rocks in sweat lodge as a soothing aromatic inviting in the good spirits. Infusion of herb used to relieve menstrual cramps and relieves cold symptoms.

Modern uses: The use of chamomile flowers is unproven (PDR Herbal Medicine, third edition). That would, of course, make the traditional uses of pineapple weed suspect. Regardless, chamomile is widely used topically to treat abrasions, inflammations, eczema, and acne with varied success. One study suggests azullene in chamomile may stimulate liver regeneration. British scientists purport chamomile stimulates infection-fighting macrophages and B-lymphocytes of the human immune system. Commercial preparations in lotions and ointments used as antiseptic treatment of sore gums, wounds, raw or sore nipples, and other inflammations. Chamomile is applied topically to treat inflammation associated with hemorrhoids (Singh, 2011).

Warning: Like many herbs, there is a paradox here; although antiallergic for some, chamomile may be allergenic to others, even anaphylactic to a few. If allergic to ragweed, best avoid using this plant externally or internally. Reports say a few people get skin rashes and allergic stomachaches from drinking or applying chamomile-containing products and cosmetics. If you have a ragweed allergy, you may also get an allergic reaction from chamomile tea.

Notes: A pineapple weed or chamomile bath (1 cup flowers in a pair of pantyhose) makes an emollient, moisturizing skin wash. Inhaling the steam may relieve upper respiratory infection (sinusitis). In an 8-quart pan mix ¼ cup fresh flowers in 1 quart of water just off the boil. Drape a towel over your head, lower head to water, and inhale for sinus congestion. Washing hair with the tea improves quality and sheen.

Corn

Stigmata maydis, L. (N.O.: Gramineae)

Identification: Corn is a member of the grass family, the genus Zea, and the species Mays. Its scientific name is Zea Mays. The common Indian corn is generally believed to have originated in the New World, where it was cultivated before Christopher Columbus discovered America. Columbus took it to Spain and many thought it was brought from Asia and it was frequently known as Turkey corn, or Turkey wheat. The silk should be taken when the corn will shed its pollen. The active principle is maizenic acid.

Solvents: Water, dilute alcohol.

Medicinal Part: The green pistils.

Effects: Diuretic, Demulcent, Alterative.

Uses: So well-known and yet not recognized by most for its medicinal properties. Herbalists and naturopaths use corn silk when dangerous deposits of brick dust are present in the urine and for removing the condition which is responsible for the disturbance in cystic irritation due to phosphatic and uric acid build up. Stigmata maydis will assist all inflammatory conditions of the urethra, bladder and kidney, which is the cause of much local and general malfunction of the body due to uric acid retention.

Dose: Tincture of Corn silk (Stigmata maydis) 15-30 drops, tincture of Agrimony (Agrimonia eupatoria) 10-30 drops, in water between meals and at bedtime. For more severe urinary complaints combine 4 oz. of corn silk, 2 oz. of dandelion root (Leontodon taraxacum), 1 oz. of golden seal (Hydrastis canadensis)_ Steep 1 teaspoonful to 1 cup of boiling water. Take every three or four hours or as needed. Sweeten with honey to taste.

Cranberry

Ericaceae *(Vaccinium oxycoccus L.)*

Identification: Dwarf evergreen shrub 5" to 15"
inches tall, but more likely a low-lying creeper
weaving its way through bogs on slender stems. Bark
hairy to smooth, brown to black in color. Flowers
pink; solitary or in couplets, rarely three; nodding,
with petals sharply bent backwards like shooting
stars. Fruit color ranges from pink to red, depending
on ripeness. Small berries are juicy and very tart.

Habitat: Nationwide in the upper tier of states. Along
the floor of sphagnum bogs, in hummocks and wet
alpine meadows to elevations of 6,000 to 7,000 feet.

Solvents: Water, dilute alcohol.

Medicinal Part: The bark.

Effects: Antispasmodic, Nervine, Tonic, Astringent,
Diuretic.

Traditional uses: The berries and berry juice were
used as therapy for urinary tract infections—they were reported to acidify urine. Some claim
that cranberry helps remove kidney stones. The juice was also used to treat bladder infections
and to prevent recurrence of urinary stones. It contains vitamin C and prevents scurvy.
Many tribes use the fruit for food.
First Nations like the Mohawk and the Inuit peoples, in what is now Canada, also used it as a
medicine; they made a poultice of the fruit to ease sore eyes and drank tea made from
cranberries to treat urinary tract infections. Its astringent properties helped reduce swelling
and tighten and tone irritated mucosal tissue, both internally and externally; this treated a
number of conditions, from infected wounds to ulcers. Tribal women made a tea of the bark to
ease discomfort during their menstrual cycles.
First Nation tribes drank tea brewed from the berries to reduce the swelling and discomfort in
glands when they had the mumps.

Modern uses: A study showed drinking the juice may prevent adhesion of Escherichia coli to
the linings of the gut, bladder, and urinary tract, thus preventing the bacterium from
multiplying and inducing disease. In another study 16 ounces of cranberry juice was shown to
be 73 percent effective against urinary tract infections. A double-blind placebo-controlled
study in 2004, however, showed cranberry supplements in pill form as ineffective against
urinary tract infections (Linsenmyer et al., 2004). Cranberry juice also functions as a urine
acidifier. Cranberries and cranberry juice are used to decrease the odor and degradation of
urine in incontinent patients. In one small study 305 grams of cooked cranberries proved
effective in decreasing pH from 6.4 to 5.3. In other tests juice showed little effect on ph.
However, there is evidence that using the concentrated (no sugar added) juice with antibiotics
may help suppress urinary tract infections. I have taken 1 ounce of the 100 percent extract in
6 ounces of water and effectively relieved a urinary tract infection. Of course, this may or may

not work for you. The required amount of cranberries or cranberry extract to treat bladder infections and stones has not been established. Seek consultation from your holistic health-care professional.

Dandelion

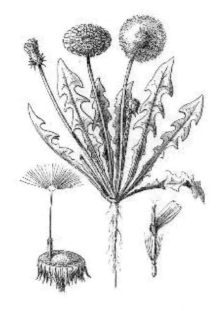

Asteraceae (Taraxacum officinale G.H. Weber ex Wiggers)

Identification: Perennial herb with a basal whorl of toothed leaves and yellow composite flower with numerous rays. Taproot is deep and bitter. Torn leaf and/or flower stem will exude white latex.

Habitat: Common yard bounty also found in meadows, along trails, and waste ground in temperate regions worldwide.

Food: A vitamin- and mineral-rich salad green. Tear it into small pieces (leave out tough veins) for salad and mix with thyme, fennel, and nasturtiums, along with other salad greens. Thyme and fennel balance the bitterness from dandelions. Make a mineral-rich tea from roots and leaves. Gently simmer chopped fresh roots for a stomach bitters. Cook fresh leaves early in season with olive oil, bacon, and lemon juice. As season progresses bitterness of leaves increases. Pour copious amount of water on the late summer plants; the morning harvest will be sweeter. Even when bitter, leaves are a healthy addition to stir-fry. Try with tofu. Cook in oyster oil, with cayenne, garlic, and beef strips.

Medicinal Part: The root.

Solvents: Boiling water, alcohol.

Effects: Diuretic, Tonic, Stomachic, Aperient, De-obstruent.

Traditional uses: The root decoction is a liver-cleansing tonic that aids digestion and helps cleanse the blood. It is also diuretic, and traditionally used to treat PMS. It has a mild laxative effect and may relieve inflammation and congestion of gallbladder and liver. Native Americans applied steamed leaves (poultice) to stomachaches. Greens considered a tonic blood purifier. Root decoction imbibed to increase lactation. Also root decoction used as mild laxative and for dyspepsia.

Modern uses: Commission E–approved for treating dyspeptic complaints, urinary infections, liver and gallbladder complaints, and appetite loss. Root extract may lower cholesterol and blood pressure (hypotensive). Dandelion is one of the most potent diuretics, performance equal to prescription pharmaceutical Furosemide in animal studies. Dandelions are a stimulating tonic and mild laxative with blood glucose regulating capacity (according to the World Health Organization, WHO). The bitter taste of dandelion is an appetite stimulant and stimulates the entire digestive system (cholagogue) improving appetite and may be helpful treating anorexia (according to the National Institutes of Health, NIH). It raises hydrochloric acid, a digestive acid in the stomach, improving calcium breakdown and absorption, and it also spurs bile production (CM).

Dose: Of the tincture 5-40 drops. For infusions, fill a cup with the green leaves, add boiling water, steep 1 hr. or longer. Drink when cold, three or four times a day. Or add 1 teaspoon of the cut or powdered root to 1 cup of boiling water and steep 1 hr. Drink cold three times a day.

Cholesterol Lowering Ability: Dandelion and other bitter high-fiber greens can theoretically lower cholesterol in three ways: 1. Stimulate the secretion of bile into the stomach, requiring more production of bile from cholesterol. 2. Fiber in the plants locks up bile in the digestive tract, preventing cholesterol emulsification, thus less cholesterol is absorbed. 3. Fiber removes bile from body, requiring the liver to break down more cholesterol to make more bile. These factors may help prevent atherosclerosis, reduce stroke, and lower blood pressure.

Possible Cancer Fighter: Researchers in Canada are studying how effective dandelion root is in fighting cancer. Siyaram Pandey, a biochemist, and his associates at the University of Windsor are studying the anti-cancer potential of dandelion root extract. His team with two years of work behind them have finished the first phase of research, showing that dandelion root extract forced a very aggressive and drug-resistant type of blood-cancer cell (chronic monocytic myeloid leukemia) to die. The team discovered that repeated low doses of dandelion root extract were effective in killing most of the cancerous cells (CBC News).

Notes: Eight plants under lights or in a window provide ample edible leaves for two people. You can eat dandelion greens and make root tea year-round. Bring plants indoors for the winter. In southern latitudes the plant is available in the yard year-round. Late-season bitter leaves can be chopped and added to salads. Flower petals may be sprinkled over salads, rice dishes, vegetable dishes.

Devil's club

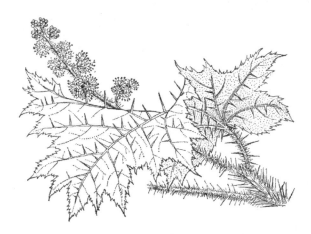

Aralioideae (*Oplopanax horridus* Sm. Torr. & Gray ex Miq)

Identification: Devil's club is a member of the ginseng family. The stems grow from 6 inches to 12 feet in height and are usually an inch or less in diameter. They possess frightening needle-sharp thorns that literally cover most of the exterior of the stem. Imagine a cane pole with thousands of steel needles protruding from the shaft and you will have a clear picture. The plant grows upright until its height becomes too much for the root and then it falls over, new roots forming along its length. The recumbent stem remains perhaps five inches above the forest floor. The wood has sweet smell. Berries shiny bright red, flattened.

Habitat: The plant grows primarily in the northwest States. The plant prefers dark and moist old-growth forest where it is difficult to see. Most people find devil's club for the first time when walking through such a forest: suddenly they find themselves tripping over a recumbent stem and falling headlong into a patch of the herb, something like falling into a Stephen King vision of a demon blackberry patch.

Medicinal Part: The bark of the root, less often the whole stem.

Solvents: Boiling water, alcohol.

Effects: Hypoglycemic, Tonic, Hypertensive.

Traditional uses: Native Americans burned devil's club, then mixed the ashes with grease to make a black face paint that was said to give a warrior supernatural power. Bella Coola Indians used the spiny sticks as protective charms. The scraped bark was boiled with grease to make dye. Native American hunters sponge a decoction of the plant's bark over their bodies to remove human odor.

Modern uses: German clinical trials show the plant has anti-inflammatory and analgesic activity. Animal studies show that a methanolic extract of the roots reduces blood pressure and heart rate (Circosta et al., 1994).

Dose:

Notes: Eight plants under lights or in a window provide ample edible leaves for two people. You can eat dandelion greens and make root tea year-round. Bring plants indoors for the winter. In southern latitudes the plant is available in the yard year-round. Late-season bitter leaves can be chopped and added to salads. Flower petals may be sprinkled over salads, rice dishes, vegetable dishes.

Echinacea

Asteraceae *(Echinacea purpurea L.* Moench*; E. angustafolia* DC*)*

Identification: Erect perennial 3' in height. Purple blossoms are large to 3" and solitary with rays spreading from umbrella shaped to flat. The bracts are rigid with thorn-like tips. Leaves are large, opposite or alternate, with smooth margins and rough surface. Rhizome (root) when sliced shows a yellowish center flecked with black, covered in a thin barklike skin. Also known as purple coneflower.

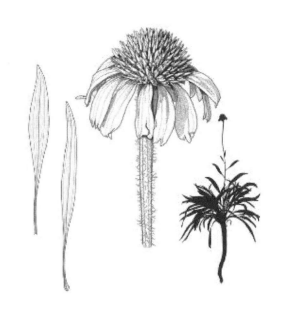

Habitat: Found in eastern and central United States, meadows and prairies, fringes of fields and parks. Cultivated in gardens nationwide. It grows throughout Arkansas, Texas, Montana, Wyoming, New Mexico, Kansas, and Nebraska, and occasionally in Colorado.

Medicinal Parts: Dried rhizome, root, leaves, and flowers.

Solvent: Alcohol.

Effects: Diaphoretic, Sialagogue, Alterative.

Traditional uses: Root and flowers used as a snakebite treatment. Boiled root water used to treat sore throats. Mashed plant was applied to wounds, and as a therapy for infections. Root infusion once considered a treatment for gonorrhea. Masticated root was held on sore tooth to treat infection. Bear-with-White-Paw, a Lakota healer, used echinacea as one of his principal medicines. He used it for tonsillitis, pain in the bowels, and toothache.

Modern uses: Commercial preparations of roots, leaves, flowers are used to treat colds, flu, coughs, bronchitis, fever, urinary infections, inflammations of the mouth and pharynx, weakened immune function, and wounds and burns. Clinical research in 2015 reports that a proprietary combination of a concentrated Echinacea herb and root extract is as effective as the conventional antiviral medicine oseltamivir (Tamiflu) when used early in the treatment of influenza (Raus et al., 2015).
Echinacea considered possibly effective at the onset of upper respiratory infections if started immediately, taken three times a day, and continued until the person is well. Echinacea aerial parts and root extractions enhance immunity in several ways. Polysaccharide-initiated response follows a bell curve: steep initial activity, improving immune response up to 32 percent. Then response peaks, and after four to six days tapers off. Therefore, it is used for acute instead of chronic conditions.
Also used internally for skin diseases, fungal infections (both candida and listeria) and slow-healing wounds, boils, gangrene, upper respiratory tract infections, sinusitis. Used externally for acne and psoriasis (not proven by this psoriasis sufferer).
Root oil has inhibited leukemia cells in vitro and vivo studies.

A recent study challenged Echinacea's immune-modulating effect (Schwartz, 2005) but subsequent studies have put Echinacea back in the news as an effective immune-modulating therapy.

Warning: A study of 412 pregnant Canadian women (206 of whom took Echinacea during pregnancy) showed malformations of babies to be equivalent between the control group and the test population, but spontaneous abortions were twice as frequent in the Echinacea group, including 13 spontaneous abortions (Chow, Johns, and Mill, 2006). As with all self-administered herbal therapies, consult your physician before using Echinacea while pregnant. The herb should be avoided by those allergic to the aster/daisy family and those with active autoimmune disease.

Dose and usage: I have prepared and used an alcohol tincture of E. purpurea flowers as a gargle for mouth and tongue ulcers. I use it to prevent colds and the flu. Commercial extracts come in solid and liquid standardized form with recommended dosage. Echinacea is also extremely useful in speeding tissue repair and in healing connective tissue. Torn ligaments respond well to echinacea and it is also of great use in healing salves for tissue repair. In combination with St. John's wort as a salve, scarring from surgery and other wounds can be reduced markedly. Echinacea is also of tremendous use in strep infections, particularly strep throat. The herb numbs affected throat tissue which helps alleviate symptoms but it is also directly effective against the infection itself. The herb should be taken as a tincture and taken by mouth.

.

Veterinarian/Wildlife: Used in pigeon racing formulas as health protecting and cleansing agent after races. Bees and butterflies flit and flip over this flower. Used in a natural product to rebuild damaged nerves in horses. Many herbalists use Echinacea to treat acute infections in pets.

Elderberry

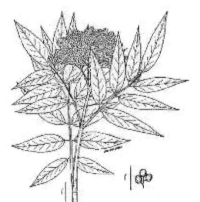

Caprifoliaceae *(Sambucus racemosa L.; S. cerulea Raf.; S. nigra L.; S. canadensis L.)*

Identification: Clump-forming shrubs. All four species have pinnately compound leaves that are opposite. S. racemosa has five or seven leaflets per leaf, green and nearly hairless above and lighter colored and hairy below. S. cerulea leaves are shiny, evergreen in the southern range; ovate or lance shaped with long pointed tips, shorter points and unequal size at base; sawtoothed edges; yellow-green color on top, paler and hairy underneath. S. racemosa has a red fruit maturing in the summer, whereas S. cerulea fruit is blue, also ripening in the summer. S. nigra (an introduced European variety and the most studied) and our native eastern variety S. canadensis are similar. S. nigra and S. canadensis grow to 25' in height. Bark light brown to gray, fissured, and flaky. Branches green with gray lenticels, easily broken. Leaves compound, leaflets oblong, ovate, serrated; matte green above, light blue-green underneath. White flowers in large rounded clusters. Fruit oval, black to deep violet.

Habitat: Nationwide. Typically in wet areas, along streams in lowlands and mountains of the West. S. canadensis is typically found in wet thickets, along edges of streams, rivers, and lakes in the eastern states and southeastern Canada. S. nigra can be purchased in nurseries and transplanted to your property.

Medicinal Parts: The roots, inner bark, leaves, berries and flowers are all recognized as natural medical treatment.

Solvent: Water.

Bodily Influence: Emetic, Hydragogue, Cathartic; Flowers: Diaphoretic, Diuretic, Alterative, Emollient, Discutient, Gentle Stimulant.

Food: Use elder flowers and berries sparingly as food because their safety is not universally established—imbibe at your own risk. We dip the white cluster of blossoms in tempura batter and then cook them like fritters. Sprinkle with powdered sugar and serve as a health-protecting, heart-stimulating dessert. Or cook elderberries, then strain the juice through a sieve, thicken with pectin, and combine with other berry jams and marmalades. The cooked juice may also be added to maple syrup. The juice mixed with brown sugar, ginger, mustard, and soy makes a good wonton dip.

Traditional uses: Flower infusions are reported to lower fever. A wash of the flowers may reduce fever and be soothing to irritations; it is considered alterative, anti-inflammatory, and diuretic. Flowers and fruit are made into tea for influenza, flu, colds, arthritis, asthma, bronchitis, improved heart function, fevers, hay fever, allergies, and sinusitis. Native Americans scraped the bark and used the root in infusion as an emetic and a laxative. The berry infusion was used to treat rheumatism. The flower infusion was given to colicky babies. Roots were pounded, decocted, and applied to swollen breasts. Leaves in infusion were used as a wash for sores.

Modern uses: Standardized extractions are Commission E–approved for treating cough, bronchitis, fevers, and colds. The therapeutic dose of flowers is reported to be 1 to 3 teaspoons of dried elder flowers to 1 cup of water off the boil. Over-the-counter elderberry extracts indicate the recommended dosage on the bottle. Flower and berry extractions are used to treat acute infections like colds and flu. Herbalist Michael Moore claims that a tincture of the flowers is alterative and diaphoretic, stimulating the body's defense systems. Elderberry flower tinctures may be more effective and more tasteful when combined with mints. The berries can act like a mild laxative, yet at the same time they are antidiarrheal and astringent. Research by Erling Thom, of the University of Oslo, presented findings on Sambucol (an elderberry over-the-counter preparation) treats and shortens flu symptoms if taken early in the episode; 93 percent of 60 patients responded positively (Thom, E., 2002).

Dose and usage: The inner, green bark and the leaves, as an expressed juice in doses of one-half to one fluid ounce, is considered reliably effective as an emetic. Lower doses will encourage gastric and fluid secretions. Because the bark is so strong, it is advisable to become informed in the use of the plant before using it too freely. Generally, the flowers and berries are most often used in conventional herbal practice. The flowers are excellent for upper respiratory inflammations such as colds, flu, and hay fever. The flower tincture (one dropperful to three times a day) will help clear mucous conditions in the upper respiratory tract, reduce inflammation, and help healing. The flowers, when steeped as a hot tea (cup of hot water to two teaspoons of the fresh or dried flowers), are considered to be a general stimulant for the body. When prepared in cold water (same proportions) they are felt to be a good laxative and effective diuretic. The berries are also often used for their laxative properties, primarily through taking a glass of the expressed juice, diluted with hot water twice a day. The flowers and leaves are often used in salves for wounds to soften the skin and help in general healing.

Warning: The leaves, bark, root, and unripe berries of Sambucus species may cause cyanide poisoning. Cook the berries before consuming them. The western variety, S. racemosa, with red berries, may be more toxic than the blue and black berries of the varieties S. cerulea, S. canadensis, and S. nigra. Avoid eating red elderberries—the fresh berry juice has caused illness.

Notes: Elderberry (fruit) may be dried in a food dryer, then frozen and used in cooking throughout the cold months for disease prevention. I eat the dried berries of S. canadensis throughout the winter on cereal, pancakes, waffles, and porridge and in stir-fries. Berries are best when cooked after drying. Flowers may be gathered in June, dried, and made into tea. Be sure to cut away the stems before eating the flowers and remove the stems from berries too.

Wild Ginger

Aristolochiaceae *(Asarum canadense L.)*

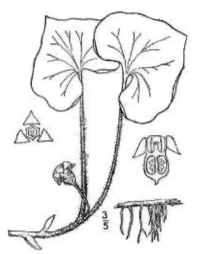

Identification: Low-lying colonial perennial herb with an aromatic root, smells like ginger; two dark-green, heart-shaped leaves. Note the hairy stem and leaves. A primitive red flower emerges under the leaves in May in Michigan. The plant grows from an adventitious rhizome and is spreading.

Habitat: Various species grow across the entire United States, except extreme desert, southern California, and lower Florida. Found on rich soil in moist woods as a ground cover in shady areas.

Food: For the daring gourmet, try boiling the root until tender and then simmer in maple syrup. The result is an unusual candy treat. Taste the leaves. Crushed root added to salad dressings. When dried and grated it is an adequate substitute for Asian ginger.

Medicinal Part: The root.

Solvent: Boiling water.

Effects: Stimulant, Carminative, Tonic, Diaphoretic, Diuretic.

Traditional uses: Root traditionally used to treat colds and cough; antiseptic and tonic. Also used in compounding traditional medicine to treat scarlet fever, nervousness, sore throat, vomiting, headaches, and earaches as well as asthma and convulsions—considered a heal-all.

Modern uses: The stimulating root considered an appetite enhancer. Herbalists use the root in tincture to dilate peripheral blood vessels, but this is unproven without double-blind, placebo-controlled studies.

Ginseng

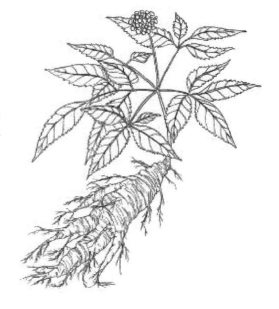

Araliaceae (Panaxginseng C.A. Meyer; P. quinquefolius L.; Panax trifolius L.)

Identification: Perennial to 3' in height. Stem smooth, round. Three to five leaves in terminal whorls with three to five palmate leaflets; leaflets, finely serrated, 3" to 8" long, 1" to 2" wide. Greenish-yellow flowers give rise to a pea-sized, rounded, glossy seed. Seeds in a cluster on a central stalk separate from leaves. Dwarf variety (dwarf ginseng, Panax trifolius) similar but smaller, to 8" to 9" tall.

Habitat: Cultivated from coast to coast, found wild in the Northwest and eastern forested areas. Rare in most of its former range. Needs shading forest with mature canopy and well-drained soil.

Medicinal Part: The dried root.

Solvent: Water.

Effects: Stimulant, Demulcent, Stomachic, Nervine, Aphrodisiac.

Traditional uses: Native Americans used the root as a ceremonial fetish to keep ghosts away. The decoction made from fresh or dried roots reduced fever and induced sweating. The root is considered a panacea in China and Korea as a tonic and an adaptogen—that is, it helps the user to adapt to stressful conditions. It is said to potentiate normal function of the adrenal gland. Ginseng root is considered a stimulant and an aphrodisiac that enhances the immune response and may improve cerebral circulation and function as well as regulating blood pressure and blood sugar. In Traditional Chinese Medicine terms, it tonifies primordial energy (increases libido). It is a tonic for the spleen and lungs.

Modern uses: Chinese, Russian, Korean, and European studies suggest that ginseng enhances production of interferon. It is considered an ergogenic aid and may improve endurance. It is reported to regulate plasma glucose. Other research focuses on its anticancer, antiproliferative, and antitumor activity against leukemia and lymphoma. Ginseng's antimicrobial and antifungal activity has been demonstrated. (Cold FX is an over-the-counter treatment for colds that contains ginseng. It has proven effective in clinical trials.) Root preparations lower or raise blood pressure. Ginseng is also used as an immune-system stimulant to help resist infection. Preliminary studies suggest it may increase mental acuity, and it has an estrogen-like effect on women. Studies suggest it may protect against radiation sickness and other physical, chemical, and biological stresses, thereby supporting its antistress applications. Considered by many the closest thing to a cure-all in nature.

Asian ginseng (P. ginseng) is considered warming and stimulating.

Korean red ginseng (different preparation of P. ginseng) warms more than Asian white.

American ginseng (P. quinquefolius) cools, moistens, and soothes.

American ginseng is considered a better tonic than Asian ginseng, at least in the eyes of Asian practitioners.

As for the performance-enhancing effects of ginseng supplements, the jury awaits more clinical trials—double-blind, placebo-controlled. So hold onto your money and follow the literature.

Dose and unse: To make a tea, take 3 oz. of powder (Ginseng 6-7 years old), add 1 oz. of honey and 60 drops of wintergreen, and blend. Use 1 tea- spoonful to 1 cup of boiling water, let it stay a little short of the boiling point for 10 min., drink as hot as you can before each meal. To make tea from the dried leaves, steep as you would for ordinary teas. Excellent for nervous indigestion.

Warning: Always use this herb under the supervision of a professional healthcare practitioner. Taking more than 3 grams of ginseng per day may cause diarrhea, anxiety, dermatitis, and insomnia. Mild reported side effects include headache and skin rash. Ginseng may strengthen the effects of caffeine. Large doses may cause hypertension, asthma-like symptoms, heart palpitations, and, rarely, dysmenorrhea and other menstrual problems. There have been two reports of interactions with phenelzine, a monoamine oxidase inhibitor. Avoid ginseng if you have diabetes, fever, emphysema, hypertension, arrhythmia, upper respiratory infections, asthma, and bronchitis. Chinese practitioners caution against using ginseng with colds (this is in contrast to its proven benefits fighting reinfection with a cold), pneumonia, and other lung infections. Do not use while on internal steroid therapy. Avoid during pregnancy and while nursing until further studies are available.

Notes: Ginseng is becoming rare in the wild. Roots may be ordered at herbs.com and from numerous other plant and seed resources. I have found many of my Chinese herbs to harbor eggs and larvae that later emerged as some exotic and startling variety of flying insects and fast-moving beetles. Ginseng roots imported from China are now sprayed with fungicide. Scrub these roots thoroughly before grinding them for use. Dwarf ginseng, pictured above, is very common in Mid-western old-growth beech/maple climax forests. It is believed the root chemistry of the diminutive plant is as effective as its bigger relative.

Use an old sausage grinder to grind hard, dried roots into powder (the dried root is tough enough to break blades of an electric pepper mill!). A typical dose is 3 grams in decoction. Simmer for thirty minutes. Or put a 60- to 100-gram root (cut to fit) in 1 liter of spirits (vodka or rum) for two weeks. Drink judiciously for its physiological effects. The powdered herb may be purchased; use 1 teaspoon of powder to 1 cup of hot water twice a day.

Goldenrod

Asteraceae (Solidago canadensis L.; Solidago spp.)

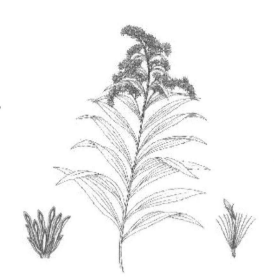

Identification: Perennial with numerous species. S. canadensis the most common eastern species, and has a smooth stem at the base, but hairy just below flower branches. Sharp-toothed leaves are plentiful, lance-shaped with three veins. Golden flowers line up atop stem, in a broad, branched spire or triangular cluster (panicle). Plant found most often in colonies. Flowers July through September.

Habitat: Nationwide fields, meadows, roadsides, railroad right of ways, vacant lots, edges of fields.

Medical Parts: The leaves and tops.

Solvent: Water.

Effects: Aromatic, Carminative, Stimulant, Astringent, Diaphoretic.

Food: Seeds, shoots, and leaves edible. Flowers made into a mild tea or used as a garnish on salads and other cold or hot dishes.

Traditional uses: First, goldenrod is not the weed that causes autumn allergies—that's ragweed—but informants say goldenrod floral tea (fresh or dried) may protect a person from allergens (hypoallergenic). Dried leaves and flowers can be applied to wounds (styptic). Traditional herbalists and pioneers used the tea to ward off acute infections like colds and flu or bronchitis, as it induces the production of mucus. Diuretic whole-plant tea is a kidney tonic. The aerial parts infused were used to treat snakebite.

Modern uses: Commission E–approved for kidney and bladder stones as well as urinary tract infections. Plants gathered when in flower and then dried are used in Europe as a relaxant (spasmolytic) and anti-inflammatory. The drug is prepared with 6–12 grams dried aerial parts in infusion. People with kidney and bladder problems should only use the herb under medical supervision. Whole-plant tea is a kidney tonic (diuretic) and may relieve nephritis (NIH) (GRIN). According to the PDR for Herbal Medicines, fourth edition (2007), the herb "has a weak potential for sensitization (can cause allergies)." Plant drug rarely causes allergic reaction.

Dose and use: 1 teaspoonful of the leaves to 1 cupful of boiling water. Externally: The Indians used the solution from boiled leaves as an external lotion for wounds and ulcers, sprinkling the affected parts with the powdered leaves as a protective dressing. The same was used for saddle sores on horses, The Spanish Americans used the fresh plant mixed with soap for a plaster to bind on sore throats. Missouri golden rod (S. missouriensis), recognized by its unusually long stemmed and fluted leaves, was eaten as salad greens.

Notes: A colorful garden addition. Also, the whole plant may be infused and used as a yellow dye.

Goldenseal

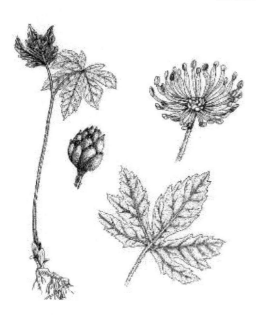

Ranunculaceae (Hydrastis canadensis L.)

Identification: Perennial to 11" in height. Bright yellow (golden) rhizome. Two ribbed leaves up to 7" wide; lower is typically smaller, sessile; upper leaf on a long petiole, with seven lobes, finely serrated. Solitary flower, found on an erect stem, with three small greenish white petals that disappear quickly. Fruit scarlet, with one or two black glossy seeds. Grows in dense colonies.

Habitat: Eastern United States. Forest dweller; wet, well-drained soil; in spreading colonies on banks in woods. Often found growing near ginseng. Cultivated nationwide.

Traditional uses: Air-dried rhizomes and root fibers were used to treat diarrhea. Cherokees used root decoction as a cancer treatment and as a tonic and wash for inflammations, infections, and wounds. Goldenseal was also used as an appetite stimulant and to treat dyspepsia. The dried root was chewed to treat whooping cough. A decoction was used for earaches. An aqueous decoction of the root was filtered through animal skin or cloth and applied as eyewash. The root steeped in whiskey was taken as heart tonic. Tuberculosis, scrofula, liver problems, and gall problems were all traditionally treated with the root extraction. According to Botanist Stephen Johnson, "The dried powdered rhizome is a good hemostat and antimicrobial that quickly forms a scab over a wound. I have used the powder this way many times with good effect."

Modern uses: Standardized extracts from air-dried rhizomes and root hairs are taken with water or in capsules to stimulate bile secretion or hydrochloric acid secretion and to hasten and improve peristalsis. The drug has a weak antibiotic and weak antineoplastic (anticancer) activity. It may constrict peripheral blood vessels and is said to stimulate and cleanse the liver. It is used as a therapy for upper respiratory infections. A few holistic practitioners still recommend it as a topical eyewash. Taken internally goldenseal may increase depressed white blood cell counts, as reported in research on Traditional Chinese Medicine. Clinical trials have suggested its effectiveness against traveler's diarrhea. The root paste is applied externally to treat wounds and fungal infections. Goldenseal's bitter taste may stimulate hunger and be useful in treating anorexia. When using over-the-counter products, seek professional advice and follow directions on the package.

Warning: Do not take goldenseal if you are pregnant or lactating due to the uterine-stimulating activity of plant alkaloids and insufficient data on breast milk and alkaloid secretions. Goldenseal is extremely bitter and may be rejected for that reason by some. It is nontoxic at recommended dosages; however, large doses of the physiologically active chemicals in goldenseal—berberine and hydrastine—may be fatal. Amounts in excess of the therapeutic dosages may cause stomach upset, nervousness, and/or depression. Large doses may cause hypertension, involuntary reflex action, respiratory failure, convulsions, paralysis, and death. The herb may negate the activity of heparin, as reported for the isolated alkaloid berberine.

Notes: Goldenseal is scarce in the wild due to overharvesting. Many botanical gardens exhibit goldenseal, and the plant is widely cultivated in the United States and Canada. Personally, I don't see goldenseal as a particularly useful herb. There are safer, more efficacious, and easier to find herbs for the same ailments. I rely more on Echinacea, Siberian ginseng, and Astragalus. I have used goldenseal for treating athlete's foot by mixing equal amounts of cinnamon, oregano, and goldenseal powder; moistening the mixture with alcohol; and then applying it with a Q-tip to areas of the foot and between the toes. My dentist's dissertation measured the antimicrobial activity of goldenseal root powder in vitro and found the alkaloids weakly antimicrobial.

Veterinarian/Wildlife: Goldenseal is one of several natural products in Brain Cool, an herbal supplement that the manufacturer claims helps rebuild nerves in horses. It is also used in training mixes, wound treatment, and fertility-enhancing formulas for horses.

Gooseberry

Grossulariaceae *(Ribes cyosbati L.)*

Identification: Sprawling or erect shrub to 5' with spiny branches with either spiny or smooth-skinned berries. Leaves alternate, deeply cleft, maplelike and long hairy petioles, three to five lobes, 1" to 2½" wide, as wide as they are long. Flowers are pale greenish yellow or white, about 4" in diameter to slightly larger, flowers tubular.

Habitat: Various species found east and west of the Mississippi as undergrowth in forests, forest edges, bog fringes, and mountain slopes.

Traditional uses: Indigenous people in North America have long used currants and gooseberries medicinally. The Comanche people used a berry tea as a gargle to soothe inflamed throats. The Prairie Potawatomi tribe made a decoction from the root, which was a good eyewash to remove foreign particles or soothe tired or infected eyes. To expel intestinal worms, the Muscogee (Creek) tribe drank a strong tea made from the root bark. Gooseberry juice was also applied to the skin as a wash to soothe irritated and inflamed skin tissue.

The berries are excellent sources of vitamin C and are rich in anthocyanins, which support circulatory health. Research is exploring whether black currant fruit shows potential to prevent liver cancer. For many years people have taken capsules of black currant seed oil (which is high in omega-3 and omega-6 fatty acids) as a dietary supplement for skin conditions, joint pain, and premenstrual symptoms.

Kiowa Indians believed that the berries would be good to treat snakebite because snakes stayed away from the plant (and seemed to be afraid of it, in fact). They would apply a poultice made from mashed berries over the bite to help draw out the venom.

Young men from the Hidatsa tribe mix clay with the red or black currant berry juice and use it as a paint to decorate their bodies for important tribal events.

Modern uses: Decoction or infusion of root used for uterine problems (prolapse). Still used by folk practitioners as an eyewash.

Gravel Root

Asteraceae (Etrochium purpureum L. La Mont; E. maculatum L.)

Identification: Perennials to 5' tall in the northern range, and up to 10' in the southern states. It grows from a rhizome on a stout stem, topped with flower heads that are domed to flat topped. Flowers are pink to purple and tubular-shaped disks. Leaves are lance shaped and in whorls, up to seven in a whorl, each leaf toothed, rough and hairy to the touch. Another species is spotted Joe-Pye weed (E. maculatum).

Habitat: Marsh, wetlands, fringes of wetlands, seeps, lakesides on damp ground, primarily eastern United States and eastern Canada.

Medicinal Part: The whole plant, especially the leaves.

Solvent: Boiling water.

Effects: Diuretic, Astringent.

Food: Not generally edible. Some American Indian tribes used the root ash as a spice or as a salt substitute and as a healing tea. Aerial parts and roots drunk as a medicinal tea to treat infections and colds.

Traditional uses: Used to treat typhus in colonial America. Native Americans used it as a revitalizing tonic to relieve constipation and as a diuretic to treat kidney stones and other urinary tract problems. Tea was used as a wash on infections to cleanse and promote healing. The root of E. purpureum was used by the Meskwakis as an aphrodisiac (they sucked on the root while wooing a man or woman). The roots of E. purpureum are preferred as medicine. The root decoction was used to treat bed-wetting in children and as a diuretic to treat congestive heart failure (dropsy).

The tea was also used for treating asthma. Native Americans used both species for treating menstrual disorders and dysmenorrhea and as a recovery tea for women after pregnancy. E. purpureum was used by Cherokees to treat rheumatism and arthritis and as a diuretic. An infusion of the root is said to be a laxative. Potawatomi used fresh leaves as a wound poultice. Navajos used the root as antidote to poisoning.

Modern uses: Hot infusions of the aerial parts are used by naturopaths to treat colds, fever, and arthritis. The plant is said to be antimicrobial and to induce sweating, loosen phlegm, and induce coughing to remove mucus. It is also used as a tonic and laxative to rid the body of worms.

Warning: This herb is no longer used with pregnant and lactating mothers.

Notes: Found in abundance in southwest Michigan but rarely harvested and used. Joe Pye, spelled historically Jopi, was a Native American healer who introduced the plant to the colonists to treat typhus fever caused by the Rickettsia bacteria. When carrying the E. maculatum species, Cherokees and other tribes used the hollow stems like straws. This plant is a striking late-summer bloomer worth adding to your wildflower garden.

Hawthorn

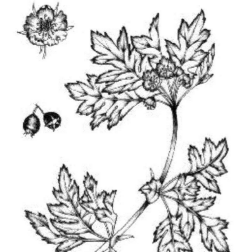

Rosaceae *(Crataegus spp.: C. laevigata [Poiret] DC.; C. monogyna Jacquin Emend.; C. oxyacantha; C. douglasii Lindl; C. macrosperma Ashe)*

Identification: Shrubs to small trees from 6' to 20' in height, many branched. Branches thorny. Yellow-green leaves glossy, three- to five-lobed, with forward-pointing lobes and serrated leaf edges. Numerous white flowers in terminal clusters, with ten to twenty stamens that give rise to small applelike fruit. Fruit ovoid to round, red or black, mealy. There is one seed in each chamber of the ovary.

Habitat: Hawthorn species are found nationwide. C. macrosperma: United States east of the prairie. Damp woods and fringes of forests. They prefer some exposure to sun.

Food: The fruit may be eaten out of hand. It's mealy and seedy, but its heart-protecting value makes it worth the trouble. The fruit may be sliced and dried and decocted or infused in water to make a health-protecting drink. It blends tastefully with green tea. Berries are gathered in August and immersed in boiling water for thirty seconds and then cut in half, seeds removed, and dried in a food dryer. Berries may be cooked in hot cereals or added to tea. Be creative.

Traditional uses: Hawthorn has long been used to treat heart disease in Europe and China. The active phytochemistry includes bioflavonoids that improve peripheral circulation to the heart and the extremities, including the brain. They also improve coronary blood flow and are hypotensive. Native Americans chewed the leaves and applied the masticated mash to sores and wounds as a poultice. Shoots were used in infusion to treat children's diarrhea. Thorns were thrashed on arthritic joints as a counterirritant. The Okanagan-Colville Nation's herbal art included burning the thorn down to the patient's skin, not totally unlike incense burning (moxibustion) on Chinese acupuncture needles to heighten effect. A decoction of new shoots was used to wash mouth sores. Numerous other remedies are discussed in Moerman's Native American Ethnobotany (Moerman, 1998).

In addition to treating physical heart conditions, hawthorn has a long history of being used for emotional well-being. The Celts believed that hawthorn would heal a broken heart. In ancient Greece, wedding processions carried hawthorn branches to symbolize hope. And in the early 1930s, Edward Bach, a medical doctor and surgeon in England, developed flower essences — a natural preparation made by steeping flowers in water and preserving them with brandy — to treat symptoms of emotional imbalance. Hawthorn flowers, in particular, were indicated for emotions of the heart.

Modern uses: Most studies have been on C. laevigata leaves, fruit, blossoms, and new end growth. Hawthorn is said to improve and protect cardiac and vascular function by dilating coronary blood vessels and initiating heart muscle regeneration. The extract may be antiangina and improve Buerger's disease (paraesthesia of foot or single toe, an arterial spasm). It's also used to treat tachycardia. Hawthorn is considered cholesterol lowering and hypotensive. The anthocyanidins and proanthocyanidin fraction are said to be synergistic with vitamin C. In European studies, use of the standardized extract improved exercise tolerance in heart patients. Other studies suggest that the extract may alleviate leg pain caused by partially occluded coronary arteries.

Chinese practitioners decoct the dried fruit and use it for treating irritable bowel and gallbladder problems. The berry is considered antibacterial to shingella (dysentery) species. A decoction of dried fruit is considered antidiarrheal and helpful in treating dyspepsia. Dr. Ann Walker, University of Reading, in the United Kingdom, published in the British Journal of General Practice a human study, placebo controlled, using hawthorn extract to lower blood pressure in diabetics. Patients taking hawthorn had a significant reduction in diastolic blood pressure but no difference in systolic pressure with no drug/herb interactions. Dr. Walker reported the blood pressure effect from the study was real (Walker, 2006).

Warning: Not recommended during pregnancy and lactation. Proanthocyanidins have been shown not to be mutagenic when tested by means of the Ames test (a standardized measure of carcinogenicity). Safety with berry extracts is well established.

Notes: Some herbs with circulation-stimulating properties, in addition to hawthorn, include garlic, ginger, ginkgo biloba extract, and cayenne. If you grow them, in the spring you can cut off a few dozen clusters of flower buds and emerging new-growth leaves to make a tea. The hot water extracts the bitter bioflavonoids that are hypotensive and anti-angina.

Heal-all

Lamiaceae *(Prunella vulgaris L.)*

Identification: Perennial typically 6" to 10" tall. Square stem erect when young; may fall and creep. Leaves ovate to lance shaped, margins dentate (toothed) to entire, and opposite. Blue to violet bract of flowers clustered in a whorl at end of square stem. Also known as self-heal.

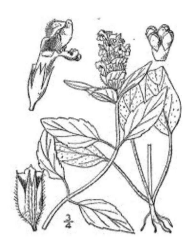

Habitat: Nationwide. Waste ground, lawns, edges of fields, margins of woods, wetlands.

Food: According to Moerman (Moerman, 1998), the Cherokees cooked and ate small leaves. The Thompson First People made a cold infusion of the aerial parts and drank this as a common beverage. Leaves and flowers may be added in judicious amounts to salads.

Traditional uses: Documented as used by the Chinese for more than 2,200 years, self-heal was used for liver complaints and improving the function of the liver. The whole plant was used in infusion to stimulate the liver and gallbladder and to promote healing. It is considered alterative; that is, capable of changing the course of a chronic disease.

Modern uses: Heal-all is still used internally by holistic practitioners to treat excessive menstruation and externally to treat burns, cuts, sores, and sore throats. The whole plant is infused and gargled for ulcers of the mouth and throat. The tea is made with 1 teaspoon of the dried whole aerial parts of the plant to 1 cup of water as a remedy for diarrhea and unspecified gynecological disorders. Consult with a professional holistic health-care professional for specific formulations and applications. Extracts of the herb are used in a dentifrice to treat gingivitis (Adamkovaa, 2004).

Notes: Locate this plant to your garden so you have it on-site and handy when you need it.

Honeysuckle

Caprifoliaceae *(Lonicera japonica Thunb)*

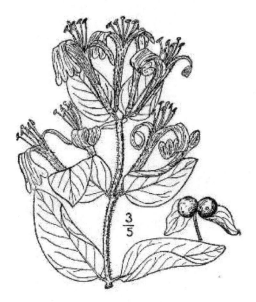

Identification: Numerous species. Shrublike or climbing vines. Elegant flowers, trumpetlike, white to off white, other species red. Leaves green, glabrous, oblong to 2" in length. Fruit is black, spherical berry.

Habitat: Fringes of woods, invasive along trails and edges of streams. Likes to border woods and not stand alone. Can colonize and become predominant invasive species in areas of development or waste ground.

Traditional uses: American species, *L. dioioa, L. canadensis* Bartr. ex Marsh, were all used by Native Americans: Floral tea used to treat dysentery, acute infections such as flu, colds, laryngitis, enteritis. The tea is antimicrobial. Tea also applied externally as a wash for edema, boils, scabies, breast cancer. Also used by First People as a blood purifier. These traditional uses suggest antimicrobial properties of bark infusion for treating syphilis, gonorrhea, urinary infections.

Modern uses: Flower extracts may lower cholesterol. Chemical extracts from leaves are anti-platelet-aggregating, perhaps preventing strokes (unproven). Saponins in the plant are anti-inflammatory.

Warning: Contact with hops and its pollen has caused allergic reactions. Fertilizers and pesticides have been eliminated as the cause—the dermatitis is caused by the plant.

Hops

Cannabaceae (Humulus lupulus L.)

Identification: Climbing perennial with pencil-thick stems that do not turn woody. The plant climbs through and atop shrubs and spreads to 30'. Leaves are opposite, three to five lobed and serrated. Male flowers are small and inconspicuous, yellowish green. Female flowers have numerous florets and a fruit cone grows from the flowers. Cone may be yellowish to gray depending on whether it is fresh or dried. The scales of the cone contain the bitter drug.

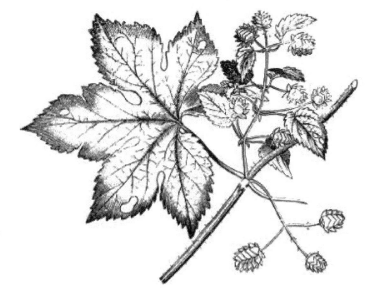

Habitat: Plant has escaped from cultivation and can be found in marshes, meadows, and the edges of woods. Cultivated stands are in northeastern Washington State, east of Seattle in the Okanagon of Washington and Canada, including northern Idaho.

Medicinal Parts: The strobiles or cones.

Solvents: Boiling water, dilute alcohol.

Effects: Tonic, Diuretic, Nervine, Anodyne, Hypnotic, Anthelmintic, Sedative, Febrifuge.

Traditional uses: Pioneers put hops in a pillow for a sleep aid. Water extraction used as a calming tea.

Modern uses: Commission E–approved for treating nervousness and insomnia (sleep aid). The flavonoids in the plant in animal and in vitro studies show them to be antibacterial, antifungal, and antitumor. Like so many plant teas, it is a diuretic. In mouse studies, humulon reduced the average number of tumors in cancer-induced mice. In another human study, hops, combined with valerian, balm, and motherwort, improved sleep in alcoholics (Widy-Tyszkiewica and Schminda). A randomized double-blind study investigated the sedative effects of a phyto-therapeutic containing valerian, hops, balm, and motherwort (Morin, 2005). The University of Chicago is completing a study of hops as a sleep aid. Related research suggests that the use is "relatively safe and effective" in inducing sleep. Early research suggested that the hop flower tea may impart estrogenic effect; subsequent research has not shown this effect.

Warning: Contact with hops and its pollen has caused allergic reactions. Fertilizers and pesticides have been eliminated as the cause—the dermatitis is caused by the plant.

Notes: For steam bath, place leaves in a clean pair of pantyhose, tie off, and put in hot bathwater. Or make a sweat lodge from a dome tent, cover the tent with a tarp and a blanket, and then heat stones over an outside fire until hot. Place stones in a large container (five-gallon enameled metal) and transfer to the floor of the tent. Place the metal tub on boards so as not to burn the tent floor. Drop water-soaked cedar boughs and hops on the hot stones, and use a long-handled ladle to dip water carefully over the rocks. Resultant steam will warm the lodge with healing aromatics. According to some sources smoking hops may provide a mild sedative effect. To make a sleep aid, add about 1 teaspoon of dried flowers to a 6-ounce cup of hot water, just off the boil. Cover, cool, and drink.

To improve cheap, watery beer place two hops into the open can or bottle and drink. Ahhh, that's better.

Veterinarian/Wildlife: Dogs have perished in as little as six hours after eating hops. Keep hops away from pets and don't drink beer with your dog.

Horsetail

Equisetaceae (Equisetum hyemale L.; E. arvense L.)

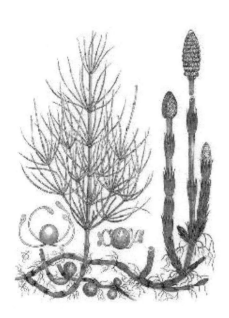

Identification: Perennial to 3' or 5' in height. Appears in the spring as a naked segmented stem with a dry-tipped sporangium (spores may be shaken from it). Later the sterile-stage stem arises, with many long needlelike branches arranged in whorls up the stem. Also known as scouring rush or equisetum.

Habitat: Nationwide. Around marshes, fens, bogs, streams, lakes, rivers.

Medicinal Parts: The leaves and root.

Solvent: Water.

Effects: Anodyne, demulcent, astringent.

Food: Native Americans of the Northwest eat the tender young shoots of the plant as a blood purifier (tonic). The tips (strobili) are boiled and eaten in Japan. Mix them with rice wine vinegar, ginger, and soy and enjoy. The roots are eaten by Native Americans in the Southwest.

Traditional uses: Mexican Americans use the dried aerial plant parts of horsetail in infusion or decoction to treat painful urination. Equisetonin and bioflavonoids in the plant may account for its diuretic effect. Native Americans used a poultice of the stem to treat rashes of the armpit and groin. An infusion of the stem was used by the Blackfoot Indians as a diuretic. Cherokees used the aerial-part infusion to treat coughs in their horses. An infusion of the plant was used to treat dropsy, backaches, cuts, and sores. Baths of the herb were reported to treat syphilis and gonorrhea. This isone of the First Peoples' most widely used herbs.

Modern uses: Commission E–approved externally for wounds and burns and internally for urinary tract infections and kidney and bladder stones. Available over the counter.

Warning: An overdose of the herb may be toxic. Use only under the supervision of a skilled holistic health-care professional.

Notes: As a fast-spreading garden plant, it does well in the shade or sun and makes an interesting addition to a flower arrangement, albeit a wandering denizen traipsing here and there through your garden. Use the stems to clean pots and pans when camping because it is high in silica.

Veterinarian/Wildlife: Ingestion of horsetail by grazing animals has caused weight loss, weakness, ataxia, fever, and other symptoms. The Meskwaki peoples fed the plant to wild geese and claimed it fattened them within weeks.

Juniper

Cupressaceae (Juniperus communis L.; Juniperus osteosperma [Torr.] Little)

Identification: Evergreen tree or lowlying spreading shrub; often grows in colonies. Leaves evergreen, pointy, stiff, somewhat flattened, light green; whorls of three spreading from the branches. Buds covered with scalelike needles. Berries blue, hard, emit a tangy smell when scraped, and impart a tangy flavor—a creosote-like taste. Male flowers are catkinlike with numerous stamens in three segmented whorls; female flowers are green and oval, fruit ripens to blue, edible, aromatic, with one or more seeds.

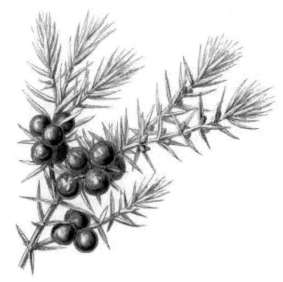

Habitat: J. communis is found nationwide, J. osteosperma found in dry montane areas of southwest and Wyoming.

Medicinal Part: The ripe dry berries.

Solvents: Boiling water, alcohol.

Effects: Diuretic, Stimulant, Carminative.

Food: Dried berries are cooked with game and fowl. Try putting them in a pepper mill and grating them into bean soup and stews and on lamb, goat, venison, duck, and turkey. The berries may be made into tea—simply crush one or two berries and add them to water just off the boil. Gin, vodka, schnapps, and aquavit are flavored with juniper berries. Use berries in grilling marinades. Grate berries on cold cuts and on vegetated (soy) protein cold cuts, like Wham and Gardenburgers. Be judicious; large amounts of the berry may be toxic (as are large amounts of pepper and salt), so use in small amounts like a spice.

Traditional uses: The diluted essential oil is applied to the skin to draw and cleanse deeper skin tissue. It has been used to promote menstruation and to relieve PMS and dysmenorrhea. Traditional practitioners use 1 teaspoon of berries to 1 cup of water, boil for 3 minutes, let steep until cool. A few practitioners add bark and needles to the berry tea. The berry is considered an antiseptic, a diuretic, a tonic, and a digestive aid. It's strongly antiseptic to urinary tract problems and gallbladder complaints but contraindicated in the presence of kidney disease.

Modern uses: Commission E–approved for treating dyspepsia. One tenth of a milliliter of the essential oil used to treat dyspepsia. The berry is diuretic, so the extract is diuretic (Odrinil). It's possibly indicated for treating heart disease, high blood pressure, and dropsy. The berry extract is used in Europe to treat arthritis and gout. Animal studies of the extract in various combinations showed anti-inflammatory and anticancer activity, but this is not proven in humans. It decreased glycemic levels in diabetic rats. In human trials the berry extract combined with nettle and yarrow extracts failed to prevent gingivitis. In one double-blind, placebo-controlled study, juniper oil and wintergreen oil (30 milliliters of Kneipp-Rheumabad) were added to bath water and reduced pain in trial participants. Mice trials suggest the berry extract in pharmaceutical doses to be anti-inflammatory, at least in the rodents. Juniper oil has been used successfully as a diuretic and may be useful as adjunct therapy for diabetes.

Dose: To make an infusion, several tablespoonfuls of the berries are generally prepared by macerating (softening by soaking), then adding them to 1 pint of boiling water for 1 hr or more. Cool and divide the mixture into four portions, which is then taken morning, noon, afternoon and evening. Dose of the tincture, 10-30 drops.

Warning: Use juniper sparingly, as allergic reactions are possible. Pregnant women should avoid this herb because it may induce uterine contractions. It may increase menstrual bleeding. Do not use if kidney infection or kidney disease is suspected. Do not use the concentrated and caustic essential oil internally without guidance from a licensed holistic healthcare practitioner.

Notes: Juniper is easily transplanted to your garden and the wild varieties, especially the western ones, provide a windfall of fruit.

Lady's Slipper

Cypripedioideae (Cypripedium acaule Aiton)

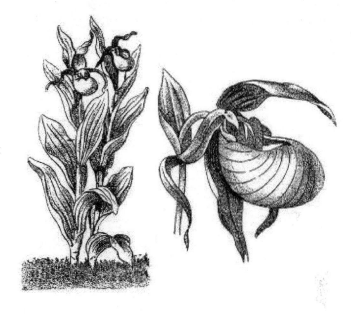

Identification: Perennial. Leaves lilylike, basal, stalkless, broadly lance shaped, to 10" in length, bright green above and pale underneath. Horizontal rhizome gives rise to orchidlike, slipper-shaped flower, typically pink, rarely white. Fruit capsule brown.

Habitat: Northern United States and Canada. Upland pine forests, wet blackspruce sites. Occasionally open wetlands. More prolific in the northeastern states and southern Ontario. Grows in profusion along the north shore of Lake Superior.

Medicinal Part: The root.

Solvents: Boiling water, diluted alcohol.

Effects: Antiperiodic, Nervine, Tonic.

Food: Not eaten.

Traditional uses: The horizontal rhizome (root) contains the active principle. It is styptic and astringent, considered a superior nervine (tranquilizer) and therefore overharvested in the wild. The rhizome was used in decoction or tincture and considered by Native Americans as a panacea for nervousness, colds, cramps, diabetes, flu, hysteria, menstrual problems, spasms, and inflammations (applied as a poultice). The rhizome is harvested in autumn and used fresh or dried for later use. Following the Doctrine of Signatures, this plant was once considered one of nature's finest aphrodisiacs because of the flower's shape.

Modern uses: This plant has been overharvested and is now protected, so its legal use has been discontinued. Its chemical constituents have not been tested but are still used to treat anxiety and insomnia.

Warning: Contact with pink lady's slipper may cause contact dermatitis.

Notes: During Memorial Day weekend, Lake Superior Provincial Park on Lake Superior is ablaze with pink lady's slippers. Bring your kayak. There are lady's slipper-studded islands just a stone's throw offshore. The species is widely protected from illegal harvesting.

Veterinarian/Wildlife: Lady's slippers are difficult to relocate because of a complex symbiosis with soil fungi. Bees, moths, butterflies, gnats, and mosquitoes pollinate the orchids.

Lemon balm

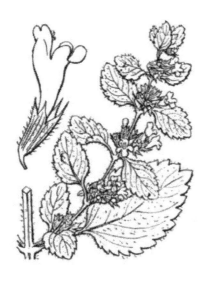

Lamiaceae *(Melissa officinalis L.)*

Identification: An aromatic many-branched perennial to 3" tall producing small white two-lipped flowers, on the end of an upcurved tube-like corolla, flowers localized in one-sided false whorls in the upper axils of the lemon-fragrant leaves. Seeds are nut brown. Stems erect, square, hairy to hairless; leaves are 3" long with short petioles and are oval to rhomboid shaped and plentiful. Lemon-scented to the touch. Blooms in summer. Also called balm melissa.

Habitat: Garden plant that escapes from garden to garden; ask your herb-growing friend to show you this plant. Feral varieties escaped to roadsides, waste ground. Widely available at garden stores; worth having.

Medicinal Part: The aerial parts.

Solvents: Boiling water, alcohol.

Effects: carminative, sedative, diaphoretic, febrifuge, antidepressant, mild analgesic, antispasmodic.

Food: Flowers and leaf buds in salads, desserts, toppings, or cooked with vegetables. Mature, aromatic balm leaves are used in baths, to make tea, and infused to flavor ice cream. A cold infusion made with other mints is excellent: Stuff a jar with all kinds of mint leaves and lemon balm leaves. Add thyme leaves and two slices of lemon. Put in refrigerator overnight. Thyme leaves make this a must-have tea for mountaineers, protecting them from mountain sickness.

Traditional uses: Phytochemicals in lemon balm may relax muscles in the autonomic system of the digestive tract and uterus. More research is needed. In Traditional Chinese Medicine, lemon balm is cooling in the second degree, like chamomile, mint, valerian, passion flower. It is a relaxing nervine, a central nervous system relaxant and calming agent. The first leaves of spring and flowers of summer may be dried. In China 1–4 grams dried aerial parts three times per day are used to treat stress. Indicated for psychological autonomic nervous system problems (stress). This peripheral vasodilator is cooling to fevers and historically used to reduce blood pressure (unproven). Traditionally considered a longevity drug.

Modern uses: Commission E–approved for insomnia and nervous agitation. However, not to be used when pregnant or lactating, as it is considered a uterine stimulant. German studies suggest that citral and citronellal in lemon balm relax the central nervous system. Polyphenolic compounds are antiviral, used specifically on herpes simplex (cold sores).

Warning: Lemon balm may inhibit thyroid function. Naturopaths use it to treat overactive thyroid.

Notes: Aggressive garden herb, at first rewarding then a nuisance. You cannot drink enough tea to keep up with it. But you cannot live without it either.

Wild American Licorice

Fabaceae *(Glycyrrhiza lepidota [Nutt.] Pursh)*

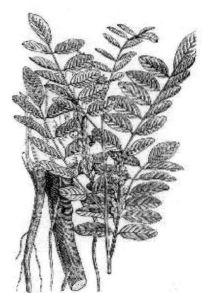

Identification: Member of the pea family with clusters of pealike flowers and compound pealike leaves. Grows in large colonies formed and connected by creeping rootstalks, which allows them to reach 5" in length. The leaves are made up of many smaller leaves along the leaf stalk (typical pea family) and are odd numbered, eleven to seventeen in number, with a single leaf at the tip. The plant stands one-and-a-half feet to three feet in height and has white to yellow-green, cloverlike blossoms. The seed pods of the plant are numerous and are a dark rusty brown and are burred, sticking easily to clothing. The burr-covered seed pods make this plant easily identifiable. The roots are the medicinal part of the plant and they are easy to harvest, growing fairly shallowly beneath the soil.

Habitat: Grows in moist, sandy soils along rivers and sunny stream banks. Ranges over the entire West and prairie states, with some extension into the East, but not Southeast. The plant likes to grow along irrigation ditches and slow-moving streams from 1,000 to 9,000 feet. It is often quite prolific when found, so harvesting an adequate supply of roots is not often a problem.

The tap roots as opposed to the runners are stronger and if you wish to spend time attacking the tough ground in which licorice grows, they may be the preferable harvest.

Taste: The American licorice is not sweet as is the European licorice. It tastes much more "pea-like." One of the benefits of the sweet variety of licorice is to make the rather strong taste of most herbal potions more palatable.

Medicinal Part: The dried root.

Solvent: Water, sparingly in alcohol.

Effects: Demulcent, Expectorant, Laxative, Pectoral.

Food: Warriors and hunters chewed the root as a sialagogue (produces saliva) to increase running endurance.

Traditional uses: The Cheyenne drank medicinal tea made from the peeled, dry roots of the plant for diarrhea and upset stomach. The Lakotas used the root as a medicine for flu. The Dakotas steeped the licorice leaves in boiling water to make a topical medicine for earache. The roots were also chewed and held in the mouth to relieve toothache. Blackfoot made a tea from roots to treat coughs, sore throat, and chest pain. They also considered it antirheumatic and applied foliage and wet, smashed roots to swollen joints. Dakota used infusion of the leaves to treat earache (Moerman).

Modern uses: Used as a flavoring agent and to sweeten tobacco. Holistic health practitioners use the herb in the same way as Asian licorice (Glycyrriza glabra) for ulcers, boosting the immune system, improving mental function, and stress reduction (no double-blind, placebo-controlled crossover studies have been done on wild licorice, G. lepidota, as of this writing).

Dose and usage: 1 lb. of Licorice root boiled in 3 pints of water, reduced by boiling to 1 quart, is an all-purpose decoction; a teaspoonful three times a day.
1 teaspoonful of the dried root to 1 cup of boiling water can be taken as an herbal tea, made fresh daily.
The root chewed raises the blood pressure in a matter of minutes.
Equal parts of tinctures of red root, echinacea, and licorice are used as an herbal flu shot of sorts. One dropperful of this mixture should be taken each hour at the onset of symptoms: it must be taken each hour to be effective.

Warning: Go gently, my friend. Glycyrrhizin in root raises blood pressure.

Lobelia

Campanulaceae *(Lobelia siphilitica L.; Lobelia cardinalis L.)*

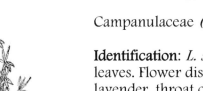

Identification: *L. siphilitica* is a perennial 3" to 4" tall. Oval leaves. Flower distinctive, birdlike, typically blue to blue lavender, throat of corolla white striped. Cardinal flower (*L. cardinalis*) has similar birdlike features but is red and not as widely distributed.

Habitat: Numerous species from coast to coast, including subalpine varieties. *L. siphilitica* is found in moist areas, streamsides, bogs, fens, wetlands of all sorts. Cardinal flower is primarily an eastern and southeastern plant, found as far south as Colombia, South America. Lobelia varieties are found from coast to coast. In western mountains the high-altitude species are much smaller in size and abundant near and above the tree line in the Sierras and the Coastal Ranges. L. siphilitica may be transplanted to a moist, semishaded area of your garden.

Medicinal Part: Leaves and stems.

Solvent: Water.

Effects: Emetic, Stimulant, Antispasmodic, Expectorant, Diaphoretic, Relaxant, Nauseant, Sedative

Traditional uses: Lobelia was used to induce vomiting and increase respiration and as a narcotic and analgesic (to treat toothache*). L. siphilitica* was used with *Podophyllum peltatum* (mayapple) to treat venereal diseases. Various species of lobelia were used for treating dysentery, cirrhosis, gastroenteritis, edema, eczema, and schistomiasis. A poultice of root was rubbed on sore neck and back muscles. Both roots and leaves were used as an external detoxifier and analgesic on bites and stings, boils, and sores. A cold infusion of the plant was considered a strong emetic. Lobelia is considered a cure for cigarette smoking, but fatalities may have occurred where the practitioner was not skilled in the use of the herb. Emetic, expectorant and nervine. The root is analgesic, anthelmintic, antispasmodic and stomachic. A tea made from the roots has been used in the treatment of epilepsy, syphilis, typhoid, stomachaches, cramps, worms etc. A poultice of the roots has been applied to sores that are hard to heal. The leaves are analgesic and febrifuge. A tea made from the leaves is used in the treatment of croup, nosebleeds, colds, fevers, headaches. A poultice of the leaves has been applied to the head to relieve the pain of headaches. Cardinal flower was used tra-ditionally in the same way as *L. siphilitica* and *L. inflata*. A few sources suggest that cardinal flower has only modest biological activity.

Modern uses: Alkaloids derived from various lobelia species have been patented. These include lobcline, lobelanidine, lobelanine, and their various salts. These patented chemicals are potential drugs in treating psychostimulant abuse and eating disorders. The drugs might be used to treat abuse of cocaine, amphetamines, caffeine, opiates, barbiturates, benzodiazepines, cannabinoids, hallucinogens, alcohol, and phencyclidine.
Cardinal flower and other lobelia species are being studied for their potential to treat nervous disorders. In a 2012 animal study published in the Asian Pacific Journal of Tropical Medicine, lobelia stopped convulsions in epileptic mice by enhancing the GABA release mechanism in the brain (Natural News, 2012).

Warning: This is a very potent and **potentially toxic** herb. Do not experiment with it.

Mayapple

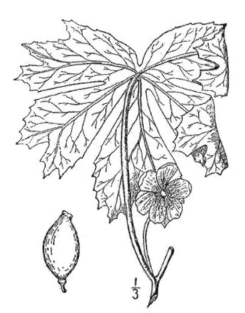

Berberidaceae (*Podophyllum peltatum* L.)

Identification: Perennial. Umbrella-like plant with cleft leaves. Leaves to 10" in diameter. Two leaves on single, stout stalk, each leaf with five to seven lobes. Single white flower tucked under leaf. Fruit ripens from mid- to late summer; edible only when ripe. Plant colonies spread over the forest floor. Also known as American mandrake.

Habitat: Extensive ground cover in eastern forests, rich woods.

Medicinal Parts: Root and resin

Solvent: Boiling water and alcohol.

Effects: Cathartic, Purgative, Cholagogue, Alterative.

Food: The fruit may be eaten in summer when it is soft and ripe. The fruit is difficult to find: Many plants die off in summer, the plants do not always provide abundant fruit (one per plant), and you are competing with forest creatures for the "apple." Cook the fruit or, if it is completely ripe, eat it out of hand. Use ripe fruit in pies, muffins, waffles, and pancakes or make it into jam or jelly. Native Americans smashed and dried the fruit as fruit cakes that were later reconstituted in water and used as a sauce.

Traditional uses: Minute doses of mayapple were used by Native Americans to treat a variety of illnesses. It treated verrucae (warts produced by papillomavirus). It is an emetic and purgative—a powerful laxative. The root is toxic and was used to kill worm infestations. Root powder was applied externally on difficult-to-heal sores. Fresh juice from the root (approximately 1 drop) was put in the ear to improve hearing. It is said that a potent extract from mayapple was used by Native Americans to commit suicide. In the mid-twentieth century, mayapple resin was injected into venereal warts as a treatment.

Modern uses: P. peltatum is Commission E–approved for treating warts, specifically genital warts. The root extract contains an antimitotic agent that led to the formulation of synthetic etoposide, a treatment for small-cell lung cancer and testicular cancer. The roots and leaves are poisonous, and handling the roots may cause allergic dermatitis. Himalayan mayapple (P. emodi) is most rich in the toxic drug podophyllotoxin.

Warning: Avoid using this plant as a drug without medical supervision. The active substance may be absorbed through the skin. It is an allergen, toxic, and antimitotic.

Gardening tip: The Menominees used an infusion of the crushed plant to kill potato bugs. Corn seeds and corn roots were soaked in a mayapple decoction to discourage fungus and other pests. I prepare mayapple root water as an insecticide for my garden. Blend about 8 ounces of fresh root in 2 quarts of water, then strain the mixture through cheesecloth or pantyhose into a garden sprayer.

Maple

Aceraceae *(Acer spp.; A. saccharum; A. rubrum; A. macrophyllum; A. nigrum)*

Identification: Crowns of trees broad and rounded in the open. Species vary in height from 30' to 150'. Bark smooth when young, furrows with age. Leaves typically three lobed. Red maple leaves have distinctive red petioles. Seeds have the characteristic helicopter-blade appearance and fly accordingly. Sugar maple leaf has the shape of the leaf on the Canadian flag. Common species include sugar maple (A. saccharum); red maple (A. rubrum); bigleaf or Oregon maple (A. macrophyllum); and black maple (A. nigrum).

Habitat: Various species broadly diversified throughout the United States and southern Canada. Wet woods, dry woods. Sugar and red maples are generally found east of the Mississippi River; bigleaf maple is a Northwest native. Black maple overlaps the range of the sugar maple in the eastern United States but is somewhat restricted to the upper Midwest.

Medicinal Parts: The inner bark and leaves.

Solvent: Boiling water.

Effects: Astringent, Deobstruent, Tonic.

Food: Maple sugar and maple syrup from the winter and spring sap are what these trees are all about. For taps or information on where to purchase them, contact a maple sugar mill near you (they'll probably sell or give you a few). Using a brace and ⅜-inch bit, drill through the bark until you hit hardwood. Clean the hole thoroughly, then drive the tap in with a hammer. Sap flows best on warm sunny days after a freezing night. In southern Michigan, tapping begins in late January and continues until early April, when the sap runs dark, thick, and stingy. Trees under 10" wide require only one tap. For larger maples you may insert two or three taps in a circle around the tree. Use a covered pail to collect the sap. If you're going to boil the sap down on an open fire, make certain your wood is dry, as smoke will give the syrup an undesirable flavor.

Traditional uses: Maple syrup is a glucose-rich sugar substitute with the added benefit of numerous minerals, a more nutritious sweetener when compared to refined white sugar. The unfinished fresh sap is considered a mineral-rich tonic. Iroquois compounded the leaves in water and drank the drug as a blood purifier. Bark infusion was used as an antiseptic eyewash. And the inner bark was decocted as a cough remedy and expectorant.

Modern uses: Maple syrup is touted as a good source of minerals, but there are no proven pharmaceutical uses as yet. Maple syrup has been used to flavor and sweeten cough syrups and has less sugar content than honey. I prefer this sweetener over others for its rich mineral content and flavor. Maple sap also contains polyphenols as well as a phytohormone known as abscisic acid, useful in helping the pancreas in its insulin production. More research necessary to prove this a viable antidiabetic chemistry (University of Rhode Island, 2010).

Milkweed

Asclepiadaceae *(Asclepias speciosa)*

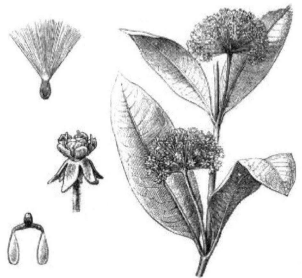

Identification: Perennial to 4' with numerous species raised on a single stem, leaves opposite, large, elliptical to 8" in length, 3" wide. Pink flowers in drooping clusters grow from leaf axils. Flowers and seedpods are striking, seedpods Arabian slipper–like. There are three main species of milkweed used in herbal medicine: the common milkweed, *Asclepias speciosa*, inmortal, *Asclepias asperula*, and pleurisy root, *Asclepias tuberosa*. While each are specific they also have certain similarities in their effects on the body.

Habitat: Edges of cornfields, waste ground, roadsides, railroad rights-of-way, meadows, dune lands, desert, and gardens. Various species found nationwide. The common milkweed, Asclepias speciosa, grows throughout the west. It is scattered and erratic but when found often grows in largish colonies. Inmortal grows primarily throughout the desert southwest and extends into western Nebraska and Arkansas.

Food: Native Americans prepared Asclepias syriaca shoots like asparagus; pick before milky sap appears, simmer in two changes of water, then sauté in oil. Flower buds are prepared like cooked broccoli when harvested before they open. Flowers buds and seedpods are prepared as follows: Boil water, pour over seedpods, let water and pods steep for five minutes, then pour off water. Repeat, pour a second boil of water over once-steeped pods, pour off water, and then stir-fry in olive oil or butter. Flowers may be dried and stored for winter use in soups, stews. Flowers have been diced, sweetened, and made into marmalade. Native Americans ground seeds into flour. You can only eat A. syriaca. Other species may be toxic. Do not experiment unless guided by an expert.

Traditional uses: Native Americans pounded or split the roots for drying. Dried roots in decoction have a mild cardiac-stimulating effect, without the toxic effects of digitalis. Be warned this should be practiced with medical supervision because Asclepias syriaca L. contains toxic cardiac glycosides and requires careful preparation before use. Native Americans believed the plant was a lactagogue (promotes milk flow) because of the milky white sap, as per the Doctrine of Signatures, or "like treats like." Latex from the leaves was also rubbed on warts, and, reportedly, on cancerous tumors. Native American lore suggests that approximately a fistful, a cup and a half, of milkweed was dried and pounded to a pulp, then mixed with three dried Arisaema (jack-in-the-pulpit) rhizomes. The plants were then put in a skin or gourd and infused into water for 20 or 30 minutes.

The infusion of the two plants was swallowed, one cup per hour, to induce sterility. All varieties were used by First People to treat wounds as a poultice. The white gum was applied over insect stings, bites, and spider envenomations. The root infusion was used for kidney ailments and the dried leaves were infused for stomach problems. Native Americans also used the white sap of the plant to treat poison ivy, ringworm, and many other skin problems. The boiled root decoction was also used externally for edema and ringworm and internally for congestive heart failure and kidney disorders. The Eclectics used dried and powdered milkweed root in a tea for asthma and as a mild sedative. According to Foster and Duke the plant is considered "dangerous and contraceptive" (Foster and Duke).

Modern uses: Homeopathic preparations are used for treating many ailments to include edema, dropsy, dysmenorrhea (as an emmenagogue). Asclepias curassavica L. from China is used to disperse fever (clears heat), to improve blood circulation, and to control bleeding. The entire plant is dried and decocted as a cardiac tonic. Other Chinese formulations are used for tonsillitis, pneumonia, bronchitis, urethritis, externally for wounds. Calotropin from Asclepias inhibits human nasopharyngeal tumors (source did not say whether this effect was in vivo, or in vitro, so take that with a grain of salt). According to herbalist Michael Moore, the dried gum may be chewed in small portions to treat dry cough, as an expectorant; the bitterness stimulates saliva flow, a potential sialogogue (stimulates saliva flow; also see sweet flag, Acorus calamus root).

Dose and usage: Milkweed is a highly useful plant. The shoots may be gathered when four to eight inches in height and prepared like asparagus. The thick, white, milky sap contains a number of cardiac glycosides and is quite bitter. The water in which the milkweed is cooked should be changed one or two times.
The root, when taken as medicine, is primarily an herb for the lungs. It softens bronchial mucous, facilitates expectoration, and dilates the bronchial passageways. As such it can find use in treatment of asthma, symptoms of colds and flu that are seated in the lungs, bronchitis, pleurisy, and chronic problems such as emphysema and cystic fibrosis.
The herb also acts well as a diuretic and increases sweating. Too much can cause nausea and, eventually, vomiting if one persists. You should start with 15 drops of the tincture three to four times a day and increase dosage until the edge of nausea is just starting to make itself apparent, then back off a bit.

Warning: Root decoction may be emetic; may stimulate the heart; and a few people may have allergic reactions to the milky sap.

Notes: Resin may be collected from leaves and stems. Cut and collect, working your way down from the top of the plant. For example, cut a leaf stem or stem near top of plant, then scrape away the white resin; when this wound dries and skins over, then cut a bit farther down and collect more resin. Collected resin will oxidize and dry in a glass or stainless-steel collecting dish. Stir or turn it occasionally for thorough drying. This process does not kill the plant as long as you leave ample growth for it to survive. Seed fiber and seed hair were used as life-jacket batting. Fragrant flowers are sweet, a potential source of sugar. The strong, fibrous stems can be made into cordage and the pulp of plant may be chopped, shredded, boiled, and prepared into paper.

Veterinarian/Wildlife: The plants are exotic-looking garden additions. They attract bees, butterflies (monarchs, fritillary) and hummingbirds. With luck you will soon see monarch caterpillars crawling over the leaves. Look out for black and yellow sucking insects called milkweed bugs (Oncopeltus fasciatus) on the underneath side of the leaves.

Mullein

Scrophularaceae (Verbascum thapsis L.)

Identification: Plants sprout a stout, tall stem from a basal whorl of large woolly leaves. Smaller leaves continue up the stem. Flowers are yellow, ¾" to 1" long, densely packed on a spike at the apex of the pole. Leaves to 15" in length, ovate, covered with gray hair; basal leaves larger, clasping upper leaves less dense, smaller.

Habitat: Found on waste ground, along roadsides, fields, railroad rights-of-way, and montane areas nationwide.

Medicinal Parts: The leaves and flower (Culpeper used the root also).

Solvent: Boiling water.

Effects: Demulcent, Diuretic, Anodyne, Antispasmodic, Astringent, Pectoral.

Traditional uses: Tea for upper respiratory-tract conditions, coughs, congestion, and infections. Used for treating bronchitis and tracheitis. Leaf and flower infusion used to reduce and thin mucus formation. Induces coughing up of phlegm (expectorant). Often combined with other expectorants: thyme (Thymus vulgaris) and coltsfoot (Tussilago farfara), for example. Native Americans made a necklace of the roots to be worn by teething babies. Decoction of leaves used for colds, and raw crushed leaf poultice over wounds and painful swellings. Mucilaginous leaves also rubbed over rashes. Said to be helpful reducing pain from stinging nettle. Dried leaves smoked to stop hiccups and to induce coughing (expectorant).

Modern uses: Commission E–approved for bronchitis and coughs. Flowers infused in olive oil are used in Europe for hemorrhoids and ear infections. Therapeutic teas are available over the counter.

Dose: Use as an antispasmodic. Pour a cup of boiling water over 1 tablespoon of dried, crushed or powdered leaf. Drink when cool.

Notes: Protect any mullein herbal preparation from heat and light. Add one or two of these plants to your yard: simply find a first year's growth, a basal rosette of fuzzy leaves; dig it out; and transplant. The next year the biennial will bloom.

Veterinarian/Wildlife: Appalachian spider bite treatment: For insect and spider bites, infuse whole fresh flowers in olive oil. Pack flowers into a small jar; cover with olive oil. Let infuse in refrigerator for at least 3 days. Apply warm oil over bite or sting every hour for 12 hours. Garlic and mullein are used as an ear oil. See your veterinarian for more detail.

Nettle

Urticaceae *(Urtica dioica L.)*

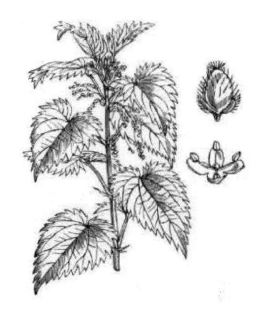

Identification: Perennial plant, erect to 5' tall with square, grooved stem, studded with stinging hairs. Leaves dark green, rough, hairy, heart- to oval-shaped, toothed; numerous green flowers borne in leaf axils, bearing numerous green seeds. Both sexes may be on one plant, or plants may have separate sexes.

Habitat: Widespread, edges of fields, streamside, wetlands, marshy areas, fringe areas, wasteland, roadsides nationwide.

Medicinal Parts: The roots and leaves.

Solvent: Boiling water.

Effects: Diuretic, Astringent, Tonic, Pectoral.

Food: Young shoots in fall (new growth) and shoots in spring are picked and steamed or sautéed. Also, stir-fry. One of my favorite recipes is to cream nettle into soup. Older summer-hardened nettles may be simmered with other herbs—rosemary, celery, thyme, onions, leeks, lovage—to make a vegetable bullion, or soup base. Discard the plant materials after simmering for twenty-five minutes. Use vegetable broth in cooking.

Traditional uses: Nettles, a mineral rich plant food, have been used for generations to treat allergies. The infusion of the aerial parts has expectorant qualities having been used for asthma and cough. Nettle tincture is used for flu, colds, pneumonia, and bronchitis. Dried plant is styptic when applied to wounds and naturopaths use the drug to treat internal bleeding. According to Brill and Dean in their book, Identifying and Harvesting Edible and Medicinal Plants, drinking nettle tea and eating nettles may make your skin clearer and healthier and it may be therapeutic for eczema. Eating nettles may improve color, texture, gloss, and health of hair. Aerial parts may be infused as a tea and used for urinary tract infections, kidney and bladder stones, rheumatism. Root tincture used for irritable bladder and prostate complaints.

Indigenous people have used nettles as medicine for centuries. The Hesquiaht and the Miwok peoples used the plant to relieve muscle and joint pain — sometimes by whipping stems of fresh nettles over the affected body areas. The formic acid contacting the skin caused a temporary burning and blistering, but it also created a rush of circulation to those parts. This improved circulation in the muscles and joints gave some lasting pain relief for conditions like arthritis. Cherokee people prepared a tea from nettles and drank it as a stomach tonic. The Cree Indians considered nettles an important women's herb during childbirth.

In traditional Russian medicine, nettle is used to treat hepatitis. Other North American plants used to treat hepatitis include lobelia, plantain, passion flower, Oregon grape, pennyroyal, dogwood, and mayapple.

In Spanish traditional medicine, nettle leaves are prepared in infusion as a diuretic, mineral replenisher, hemostat, and to purge toxins from the body (purgative). The root is believed to reduce the size of kidney stones. A decoction of the seeds is believed to prevent involuntary urination in children.

Stinging nettle is said to be helpful on arthritic joints as a counterirritant. Mexican truck drivers use the plant to relieve sciatica. They also drink copious amounts of tequila. I recommend if you use the nettle arthritis remedy, have the tequila ready. Scarification is another way that Native Americans treated arthritis. See the DVD Native American Medicine and Little Medicine available from the author.

Nettles have been used to thrash arthritic joints. Whipping the arthritic area causes pain and inflammation and temporary relief. Not recommended. However, when nettles come in contact with a painful area of the body, they actually do decrease the original pain, perhaps by reducing inflammatory chemicals and interfering with neural pain signals.

Modern uses: Commission E–approved for treating benign prostatic hyperplasia (BPH). Nettle root and saw palmetto have been combined successfully to treat prostate enlargement symptoms (Blumenthal, et. al., 2000). Nettle roots in Russia are tinctured for hepatitis and gallbladder inflammation. In Germany, as in the US, nettle root extract is being researched for the treatment of prostate problems.

A randomized study of arthritis sufferers suggests that stinging nettle extract, when accompanied by a lowered dose of the anti-inflammatory drug diclofenac, improved or enhanced the efficacy of the prescription drug. In the test, half the patients took the full, 200 mg dose of diclofenac while the test group took 50 mg of diclofenac along with 50 g of stewed nettle leaf. The results showed that the reduced prescription drug and nettle combination was just as effective at lowering pain as the full dose of the drug. These results confirmed the 1996 study of Ramm and Hansen, showing a lower amount of prescription antiinflammatory was effectively enhanced by dried nettle-leaf capsules.

Sodium formate, an analog of formic acid found in stinging nettle and ants, makes a metal-based cancer treatment called JS07 fifty times more effective than the JS07 alone (University of Warwick).

Dose and usage: A nettle tonic is strong but gentle in action. It's what herbalists call a whole-body tonic, because it supports the functions and health of every body system. It's been used in many ways, from encouraging good digestion to relieving allergies through its antihistamine actions. It finds its way into remedies for respiratory and skin conditions and to nourish the blood. Mostly the aerial parts are used, but a tea or tincture made from the roots and taken internally can support men's prostate health.

Notes: If you cannot obtain fresh nettle, then freeze-dried is your next best choice. Nettle grows readily in a garden and provides edible leaves for up to nine months. Harvest the new-growth leaves at the top of the plant and watch as the picked stem bifurcates and grows two new growth sprouts. In effect, you have doubled your crop. Try rubbing out the sting of nettle with mullein leaves or the juice of spotted touch-me-not (jewelweed, Impatiens capensis).

Veterinarian/Wildlife: Nettle juice mixed with nettle seeds is a good hair tonic for domestic animals.

Oak

Fagaceae *(Quercus spp.)*

Identification: The best way to learn to identify oaks is to visit an arboretum. There the oaks will be labeled for identification. Armed with this visual proof, you will be more successful in the bush gathering nuts for the winter. Acorns vary in size and taste. Leaves are lobed, cut, pointed, or rounded, varying by species.

Habitat: Many species nationwide. Yards or wood lots, forested areas, roadsides.

Effects: astringent

Medicinal part: Bark and oak galls, which contain the most tannins.

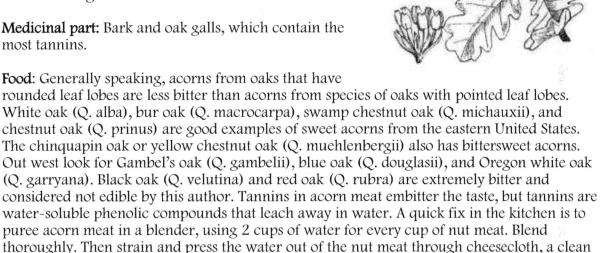

Food: Generally speaking, acorns from oaks that have rounded leaf lobes are less bitter than acorns from species of oaks with pointed leaf lobes. White oak (Q. alba), bur oak (Q. macrocarpa), swamp chestnut oak (Q. michauxii), and chestnut oak (Q. prinus) are good examples of sweet acorns from the eastern United States. The chinquapin oak or yellow chestnut oak (Q. muehlenbergii) also has bittersweet acorns. Out west look for Gambel's oak (Q. gambelii), blue oak (Q. douglasii), and Oregon white oak (Q. garryana). Black oak (Q. velutina) and red oak (Q. rubra) are extremely bitter and considered not edible by this author. Tannins in acorn meat embitter the taste, but tannins are water-soluble phenolic compounds that leach away in water. A quick fix in the kitchen is to puree acorn meat in a blender, using 2 cups of water for every cup of nut meat. Blend thoroughly. Then strain and press the water out of the nut meat through cheesecloth, a clean pair of pantyhose, or a clean white sock. I like acorn mash on baked potatoes, mixed into tomato sauces, and in all baking recipes. Also eat out of hand as a snack.

Traditional uses: Native Americans mashed and sun-dried the acorn meat before using it for food, as drying the meats makes them more palatable. White oak (Q. alba) has tannin-rich bark. Tannins are antiseptic and astringent. Native Americans and pioneers made a tea from the bark for mouth sores, burns, cuts, and scrapes. The bark extraction, considered a panacea, was believed to provide cancer protection. Dried and powdered bark was sprinkled over the navel of an infant to heal the wound caused by removing the umbilical cord. Red oak (Q. rubra) bark in decoction was used to treat diarrhea; the tannins once again account for the reported effectiveness of this remedy. The bark of pin oak (Q. palustrus) was prepared in decoction for dysentery and for edema of joints. The inner bark was heated and infused with water by dropping a hot stone into a gourd or skin bag, and the resulting tea was taken for intestinal pain (analgesic). Chinquapin oak (Q. muehlenbergii) bark was decocted by people of the Delaware and Ontario Nations to stop nausea and vomiting (antiemetic). Most species of oak bark were boiled and the decoction taken internally for dysentery and diarrhea. And the bark and wood decoction of tannin-rich oaks was used externally to treat inflammations, sores, hemorrhoids, sore muscles, and tender joints.

Modern uses: Oak bark extract, typically from Q. robur or Q. petraea, is Commission E–approved for treating bronchitis, cough, diarrhea, mouth and throat sores, and inflammations of the skin. Chemicals from oak bark are being tested as a cancer therapy.

Dose: A decoction is made from 1 oz. of bark in 1 quart of water, boiled down to 1 pint, and taken in wineglass doses. Excellent as a gargle for sore throat. Oak is often used as a strong infusion or tea for gum inflammations, skin abrasions, sunburn, bleeding wounds, diarrhea, dysentery, and hemorrhoids. One teaspoon of the bark powder in a cup of water is boiled gently for fifteen minutes and applied to the affected area.

For bleeding wounds, I have found the powdered herb (leaves, twigs, bark, or galls) to be especially effective when applied directly to the affected area. Often, I will use the oak in combination with powdered antibiotic herbs such as usnea or echinacea. Gum inflammations respond well to a tincture of the bark, other complaints respond well to the strong infusion or tea. For use in diarrhea or dysentery drink the tea, prepared as above, three to six cups a day. These conditions also respond extremely well to the use of the tea as an enema.22 Oak enemas were, at one time, a primary approach to the treatment of extreme cases of dysentery. Indian tribes are known to have allowed acorn meal to go moldy in a dark, damp place and then scrape the mold off for application to boils, sores and other inflammations.

Notes: All oak nut meats can be improved by an overnight soaking in fresh water. Native Americans would shell, crack, or smash the acorns, then place them in a skin bag and soak them in a stream for a day or two to remove the bitter tannins. Chopping the acorn meats thinly, then drying them, reportedly attenuates the bitter taste.

Oregon Grape

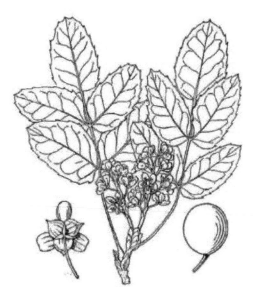

Berberidaceae (Mahonia aquifolium [Pursh] Nutt.; M. nervosa [Pursh] Nutt.)

Identification: M. aquifolium: Evergreen shrub to 6' tall. Gray stem. Hollylike, shiny leaves; pinnate, compound, pointed edges. Flower small, bright yellow. Berries deep blue, waxy. Roots and root hairs, when peeled, are bright yellow inside due to the alkaloid berberine. M. nervosa is a smaller forest dweller with rosette of compound leaves in a whorl up to 3' tall, berries on central spikes.

Habitat: M. aquifolium: Washington State east into Idaho and Montana. Along roadsides and forest edges. M. nervosa: Pacific Northwest. Along Mount Baker Highway in Washington en route to Mount Baker, in open forests and graveyards.

Food: The tart berries of M. aquifolium are eaten in late summer in Northwest. Native Americans smashed the berries and dried them for later use. They may be boiled into jam, but be certain to add honey or sugar, because the juice is tart. Carrier Indians of the Northwest simmered the young leaves and ate them. The smaller creeping M. nervosa was prepared and eaten in the same way and is preferred, but it is not as abundant. Try berries mixed with other fruit to improve the taste. Berries may be pounded into paste, formed into cakes, and dried for winter food.

Traditional uses: When eaten raw in small amounts, the fruit is slightly emetic. Tart berries of both species were considered a morning-after pick-me-up. Native Americans believed the berries were slightly emetic. A decoction of stems was used by Sanpoils as an antiemetic. These two species of bitter and astringent herbs were used to treat liver and gallbladder complaints. The bark infusion was used by Native Americans as an eyewash. According to traditional use, the decocted drug from the inner bark (berberine) stimulates the liver and gallbladder, cleansing them, releasing toxins, and increasing the flow of bile. The bark and root decoction reportedly was used externally for treating staphylococcus infections. According to Michael Moore (Medicinal Plants of the Mountain West), the drug stimulates thyroid function and is used to treat diarrhea and gastritis. According to Deni Brown (Encyclopedia of Herbs and Their Uses), M. aquifolium has been used to treat chronic hepatitis and dry-type eczema. A root decoction of M. aquifolium was used by the Blackfoot peoples to stem hemorrhaging. They also used roots in decoction for upset stomach and to treat other stomach problems.

Modern uses: M. aquifolium extractions are available in commercial ointments to treat dry skin, unspecified rashes, and psoriasis. The bitter drug may prove an appetite stimulant, but little research has been done. Other unproven uses in homeopathic doses include the treatment of liver and gallbladder problems. Three human studies showed Mahonia aquifolium skin application (10 percent cream or ointment extract from leaves and root) as effective in treating psoriasis. Each study had positive results. Participants rated the M. aquifolium extract as good as, or better than, standard Dovonex cream, an expensive prescription alternative. This is good news to psoriasis sufferers, and that includes me (Gulliver, 2005).

Warning: Do not use during pregnancy or while nursing.

Notes: The shredded bark and roots of both species was simmered in water to make a bright yellow dye.

Veterinarian/Wildlife: Berries are eaten by birds. The Saanich people claim the berries to be an antidote to shellfish poisoning. They chewed M. aquifolium for protection after hunting when approached by a dying deer. Oregon grape is an ingredient in a training mix and nervous system formula for horses.

Pasque Flower

Ranunculaceae (*Pulsitilla spp.*)

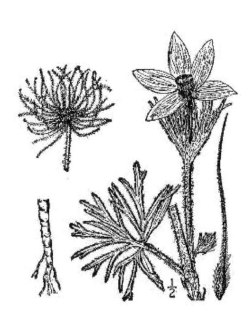

Identification: Across all thirty-three species the plant characteristics are similar: finely dissected leaves, hairy stems, and bell shaped flowers. The biggest variable is height; species range from 3" to 9". Showy parts of the flower are the sepals. Seed heads are plumed. The lilac-colored pasque flower (*Pulsitilla patens*) is covered with a soft hairy down, usually producing only one or two flowers from its small root.

Medicinal Parts: Plant and flower.

Effects: Tonic, Sedative, Nervine

Habitat: Found in the prairie and mountain meadows. Pictured specimen from the Cloud Peak Wilderness, Bighorn Mountains, Wyoming.

Food: Not edible, highly toxic. May slow heart and cause cardiac arrest.

Traditional uses: Used historically by the Blackfoot nation to induce uterine contractions leading to abortion. Also believed to speed difficult childbirth. The Dakotas call it hokshi-chekpa wahcha (twin flower). The Lakotas call it hoksi' cekpa (child's navel). Blackfeet call it napi (old man). Omaha and Ponca call it te-zhinga-makan (little buffalo medicine). It was one of the sacred power medicines of the Omahas and Poncas and esteemed very highly. Among the latter two tribes, the right to use the pasque flower was limited to the medicine men of the Te-sinde gens.

Modern uses: Used as a homeopathic preparation or in combination homeopathically for a variety of ailments to include colds, coughs, and digestive problems. The olfactory essence of the flower is used in aromatherapy and reported to relieve shyness.

Warning: May slow heart and cause cardiac arrest.

Passionflower

Passifloraceae (Passiflora incarnata L.)

Identification: There are numerous varieties, all somewhat similar. It is a perennial vine on a woody stem climbing to 35' or more. Bark is longitudinal and striated when mature. Leaves are alternate, with petioles, serrated with fine hair on both the top and bottom, but underside of leaf is hairier. Leaf blades have bumps called floral nectaries. Flowers are single, wheel shaped, petals like spokes, striking, to 5" in width.

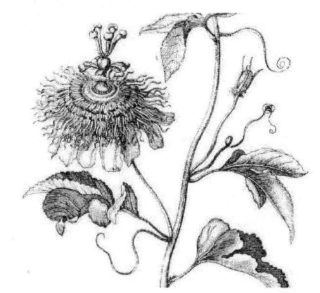

Habitat: Climbing vine of open areas and the forest edge. Most species tropical or subtropical, but will grow in a temperate garden. With a worldwide distribution, numerous species are found across seven climactic zones. Often introduced. Found wild in the southeast United States.

Medicinal Parts: Plant and flower.

Solvent: Diluted alcohol.

Effects: Anodyne, Nerve sedative, Diuretic, Antispasmodic.

Food: The leaf and flower tea has mild sedative properties. Fresh fruit may be eaten raw or juiced or made into a beverage. Mexicans mix with cornmeal or flour and eat it as a gruel. Leaves eaten by Native Americans. Typically, leaves are parboiled and pan-fried in vegetable oil or animal fat.

Traditional uses: Fresh or dried aerial parts or whole dried herb used in infusion as mild sedative. Also used to treat nervousness and insomnia—a sleep aid. Antispasmodic effect of infusion considered a gastrointestinal aid. People used the infusion of crushed root for treating earache. They also pounded root, and applied the mass as a poultice on inflamed contusions, boils, and cuts. The root water of the plant was mixed with lye-treated corn and used to wean babies. The tisane was considered a blood purifier for many tribes. Pioneers used the whole plant with Epsom salts as a sedative bath. Root tea and aerial-parts tea used for treating hemorrhoids.

Modern uses: As above. In animal studies, infusion was reported as sedative, antispasmodic, and inhibited motility of organisms. Commission E–approved for treating nervousness and insomnia. Use as an antidepressive and for treating somatization disorder (colloquial: hysteria) is unproven.

Notes: The Doctrine of Signatures suggests that this sensual-looking plant is an aphrodisiac. Passiflora contains betacarboline harmala alkaloids, which are MAOI (monoamine oxidase inhibitors) with antidepressant properties. Typically the flower has only traces of the chemicals, but the leaves and the roots of some species have been used to enhance the effects of mind-altering drugs.

Veterinarian/Wildlife: Extract is used to calm stressed cats, and has been used as a mild sedative for horses.

Peppermint

Lamiaceae *(Mentha spp.: M. piperita L.)*

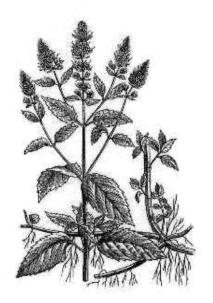

Identification: There are many American members of the mint family. Common characteristics include: square, erect stem, leaves almost always aromatic when crushed, typically aggressive and spreading. Species vary in height from 8" to 30" tall. Root a spreading rhizome. Leaves plumply lance shaped (elongated) to ovate to roundish, typically serrated. Flowers in dense whorls culminating in a terminal spike of blossoms or in clusters in the axils of leaves. Flower colors vary by species: white, violet, blue. One common species is peppermint (Mentha piperita).

Habitat: Nationwide. M. piperita can usually be found around water, shorelines, stream banks, and dunes of the Great Lakes and in or around mountain passes, blowdowns, avalanche slides, and wet meadows.

Medicinal Parts: Leaves and stems.

Solvent: Water.

Effects: Aromatic, Stimulant, Stomachic, Carminative.

Food: Peppermint is used in teas, salads, and cold drinks; with sautéed vegetables; and as an integral part of the subcontinent and Middle Eastern flavor principles. Romans such as Pliny the Elder used mint to flavor wines and sauces. Mint is excellent in Mexican bean soups or in chilled soups of all kinds.

Traditional uses: Aristotle considered peppermint an aphrodisiac, and Alexander the Great thought that eating mint or drinking the tea caused listless, unaggressive behavior. Peppermint leaves and flowers are infused in water and taken as an uplifting tea. The extracted oil (as well as the tea) is antiseptic, carminative, warming, and relieves muscle spasms. An infusion increases perspiration and stimulates bile secretion. Menthol and menthone, peppermint's inherent volatile oils, are antibacterial, antiseptic, antifungal, cooling, and anesthetic to the skin.

Modern uses: Leaf and flower extraction are Commission E–approved for treating dyspepsia, gallbladder, and liver problems. Peppermint oil is approved for colds, coughs, bronchitis, fevers, mouth and larynx inflammations, infection prevention, dyspepsia, and gallbladder and liver problems. Recent studies in Europe suggest it may be a treatment for irritable bowel syndrome. The tea and oil have an antispasmodic effect on the digestive system. Peppermint is also used to treat colic, cramps, and flatulence. It may help relieve diarrhea, spastic colon, and constipation. Headache due to digestive weakness may be relieved by taking peppermint, and trials using the extract to treat tension headaches look promising (the essential oil is diluted and rubbed on the temple to relieve headaches and tension). The diluted oil is used in aromatherapy for treating headache and as an inhalant for respiratory infections (i.e., rubbed on the chest). Enteric-coated capsules are used for irritable bowel syndrome and to relieve colon spasms during enema procedures. In vitro comparative research in 2014 found peppermint suppressed growth and induced cell death (anticancer effect) against human laryngeal carcinoma (Abirami and Nirvada, 2014). So drink your mint tea and good things may happen.

Warning: In too high a concentration, the mint oils are a skin irritant and may burn. Be careful. Peppermint is contraindicated for ulcers, gastritis, and acid reflux because it relaxes the esophageal sphincter, allowing stomach acid to escape into the esophagus (acid reflux).

Notes: Peppermint, spearmint, mountain mint, and other mints have edible flowers and leaves that may be used in salads and desserts. Try mint blossoms on sliced pears. Mint is a carminative herb used to dispel gas. For a dollar or so buy mint lozenges (Altoids) and use them to alleviate gallbladder pain and pain from a spastic colon. The mint lozenges may quell the discomfort from irritable bowel syndrome.

Gardeners beware: Grow mints in a buried steel container to prevent their unabated spread.

Veterinarian/Wildlife: Historically mint was strewn around floors as a vermifuge to rid the home of insect and rodent pests.

Pine

Pinaceae (Pinus spp.: P. strobus L.; P. edulis L.)

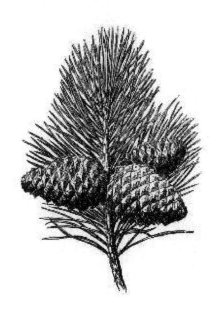

Identification: White pine (Pinus strobus) is an evergreen tree with medium to long needles. Needles in clumps of five, light green with single white stripe. Pinyon pine (P. edulis) is a stubbier plant isolated in dry alpine areas of the four-corner region north to Canada, especially abundant on the east side of Flaming Gorge, both in Wyoming and Utah. Its cones harbor the delicious pine nut used to make pesto.

Habitat: White pine: eastern United States. Pinyon pine: dry plateaus from Mexico north to Canada. Scotch pine: planted as an ornamental in yards, fencerows, and fallow fields.

Medical Parts: Inner bark or sprigs.

Solvent: Boiling water.

Effects: Expectorant.

Food: White pine needles may be made into a tea. I take a handful of needles, crush them, and add them to a gallon jar of water containing mountain mint, lemon thyme, and lemon balm. Squeeze in juice of half a lemon and let the mixture infuse in the refrigerator for six hours. Uplifting! Seeds from pinecones may be eaten. Pinyon pine provides the most notable edible seeds used in pesto.

Traditional uses: Pine sap is styptic and wound sealing and was used by pioneers and First People to treat gunshot wounds, cuts, scrapes, and lacerations. There is historical evidence that the presence of antiscorbutic quantities in pine needles helped prevent scurvy, which supports the historical tradition of drinking pine needle tea.

Modern uses: Oil from the needles of Scotch pine shoots is Commission E–approved to prevent infection and to treat blood pressure problems; colds, coughs, and bronchitis; fevers; oral and pharyngeal inflammations; and neuralgias. Most pines and firs have vitamin C in their needles, especially end needles—a wilderness way to get the tree's antiscorbutic effect.

Notes:
Pine needles made as a sun tea are a wonderful source of vitamin C and simple carbohydrates that provide fast energy. This is a good wilderness tea for backpackers, as pine trees grow abundantly in North America and so are readily available. The needles contain five times more vitamin C than lemons do by weight.
I brew a tea from all of these pines, mixed with lemon balm, mint, fennel, and lime juice. It's invigorating and anti-infective. This brew is made overnight by cold infusion. Stuff the leaves into a gallon jar, fill the jar with pure water, refrigerate for twelve hours, then drink. Pinyon pine nut ice cream, served in Guanajuato and Dolores Hidalgo, Mexico, is one of my favorite treats. Chop some pine nuts, mash them into vanilla ice cream, and let them infuse overnight. Terrific!

Plantain

Plantaginaceae (Plantago lanceolata L.; P. major L.; P. maritima L.)

Identification: Several varieties are found across the United States. The difference is in the leaves: P. major's leaves are broad and ovate, and P. lanceolata's leaves are narrow and lance-shaped. And Plantago maritima leaves are narrow, almost linear, and it is found along the West Coast, often submerged during high tide. The green flowers of all three species are borne on terminal spikes.

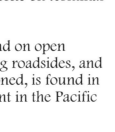

Habitat: These common plants are found on open ground, wasteland, edges of fields along roadsides, and in lawns. Plantago maritima, as mentioned, is found in the upper tidal zone especially abundant in the Pacific Northwest.

Medicinal Part: The whole plant.

Solvent: Water.

Effects: Alterative, Astringent, Diuretic, Antiseptic.

Food: In the spring, chop whole leaves into salads or sauté them with wild leeks, nettles, dandelions, and watercress. Tear the tough mid-leaf vein (rib) from summer and autumn leaves before adding them to salads.

Traditional uses: The flowering heads may be stripped off between thumb and forefinger into hot water to form a mucilaginous drink for treating constipation. A few folks believe this plant when crushed and applied is a good antidote or treatment of poison ivy. Native Americans chewed the leaves, mixing in saliva and defensin (a chemical in our mouths that is antibiotic and immune stimulating) to provide an antiseptic and immunestimulating poultice to be applied to wounds, scrapes, cuts, or bruises. Digestive enzymes in our mouths are also weakly antimicrobial, while the plantain is styptic, stopping blood flow. Simply chew the plantain leaf and fix it in place over the wound. Plantain lotions and ointments are used to treat hemorrhoids, skin fistulae, and ulcers.
Tea is diuretic, decongestant, expectorant. May be helpful in diarrhea, dysentery, irritable bowel syndrome, laryngitis, and urinary tract bleeding. Acubin increases uric acid excretion by kidneys and may be helpful in treating gout.

Modern uses: Commission E reports that P lanceolata extract from the fresh plant may fight colds (4 grams of herb to 1 cup boiling water), may alleviate symptoms of bronchitis and cough, and may reduce fever. The commission also approves the herb for treating inflammation of pharynx and mouth, and for skin inflammations. Also used in respiratory-tract infections and is considered antibacterial. The tea of the fresh leaves is used to treat respiratory-tract infections and is considered antibacterial (GRIN). Typical dose is 3–6 grams of the fresh whole herb (aerial parts when in bloom) added to 1 cup of water just off the boil. Let it cool, strain away plant material, and then drink 3 or 4 times a day.

Notes: Humans have chewed the leaves and applied the masticated mass over wounds. Plantago seeds from India and Africa are dried and used as a bulking laxative. Plantago ovata is a constituent of Metamucil.

Veterinarian/Wildlife: P. major is a favored food of the eastern box turtle. Tough leaf veins can be stripped and in an emergency used as fishing line, or even used as suture material for saving a hunting dog bitten by a bear, for example. Plantain seed, known as psyllium, is used in training mixes and wound treatment formulas for horses.

<u>Prickly Pear</u>

Cactaceae *(Opuntia* spp.*)*

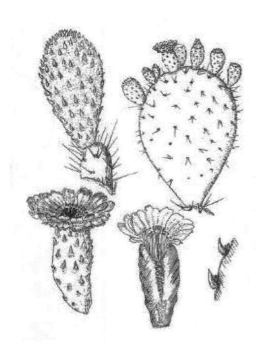

Identification: Spreading desert and arid land cactus with large oval pads (from 4" to 10") and thorny leaves of various sizes. Flowers yellowish. Fruits variable, typically white to red to purple, 2" in length and 34" wide.

Habitat: Various species found from coast to coast in dry, sometimes sandy areas and limestone hills (badlands), along roadsides in eastern Colorado, much of Wyoming, Utah, and other dry areas of western states.

Food: The pads, which are often mistaken for leaves (actually, the spines are the leaves), are edible. Most edible species have flat joints between pads. Flowers and flower buds are roasted and eaten. Species with plump pads (the new growth is preferred) may be thrown on hot coals of fire and roasted. The fire burns off the spines and cooks the interior. Let the pads cool, then peel the skin and eat the inner core.

The fruit when red and ripe is tasty and often made into jelly.

The pads can be mixed with water, sugar, and yeast and fermented into an alcoholic drink. The young green fruit is boiled and eaten by Pima Indians.

Traditional uses: The flowers are astringent and can be poulticed over wounds. Flowers prepared as a tea are taken for stomach complaints including diarrhea and irritable bowel syndrome. The stem ash is applied to burns and cuts. Pima Indians believe the edible pads are good for gastrointestinal complaints. Leaf pads are scorched of spines, then sliced in half and the moist side applied as a poultice for cleansing and sealing wounds, infections, bites, stings, and snake envenomations. The Pimas despined, cooked, sliced, and poulticed plants on breasts as a lactagogue. The infusion of stems of a Sonoran Desert species, *O. polyacantha* (plains prickly pear), was used to treat diarrhea.

Modern uses: In Mexico and the American Southwest, prickly pear is still used in its traditional ways. According to Andrew Chevallier (Encyclopedia of Medicinal Plants), the flowers are still used for treating an enlarged prostate. The inner flesh of the pad is a chemotactic attractant, a surfactant, that draws serum from the wound site, thus cleaning and sealing it. Try the fruit peeled, sliced, and eaten with a spicy dose of cayenne pepper. Prickly pear cactus (nopal fruit) contains twenty-four of the known betalains, which are potent anti-inflammatory agents. Betalains are polyphenolic pigments found in beets and nopal and other plants. The fruit juice is anti-inflammatory and hypoglycemic.

Gardening tip: This cactus transfers to the garden and is hardy and a summer supply of edible flower petals. It is good to have handy for its antiseptic and sealing properties.

Veterinarian/Wildlife: Opuntia pads are sliced open and applied, moist side down, over wounds, bites, stings, and envenomation. Southwestern holistic practitioners report success in treating scorpion and recluse spider bites.

Evening Primrose

Onagraceae (Oenothera biennis L.)

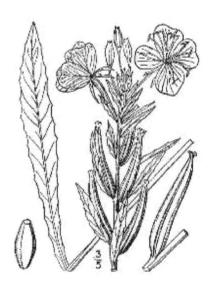

Identification: This biennial grows to 3' or more with fleshy turniplike root. First-year plant is a non-flowering basal rosette of leaves; second-year is an erect, blooming plant, conspicuous in the autumn with its large seed-filled fruit capsules. Oblong lance-shaped leaves, pointed and finely dentate. Fragrant bugle-shaped yellow flowers, 1" long growing from the leaf axils. Flowers open in evening. Fruit is linear-oblong, 4 sided, downy, about ½" to 1" in length, containing dark gray to black seeds with sharp edges.

Habitat: Found in gardens, along roadsides, on waste ground, fields, and prairies nationwide.

Food: The root is edible (biennial plant: first-year root best). New leaves of first or second year edible in salads, stir-fry. The leaves are tough and need to be cooked. Seeds can be poured out of seed capsule (seed capsule looks like small dried okra pod). Immature seed capsules may be cooked like okra, but do not taste like okra.

Traditional uses: Native Americans used warm root poultice to treat piles. Roots were chewed to increase strength and endurance. Whole plant bruised, soaked, and used as a poultice on bruises and sores.

Modern uses: The seed oil is used to treat essential fatty-acid deficiency and to lower cholesterol. Cholesterol-lowering effect was not effective in a 1986 study but did prove successful in a double-blind crossover study conducted in 1994 (Guivernau, Meza, Barja, et al.). Seed extract said to dilate coronary arteries and clear arterial obstruction. Used as a holistic treatment for intermittent claudication. Other uses include treatments of atopic eczema and psoriasis (not effective with this author). Oil may provide relief from premenstrual syndrome (PMS) symptoms, although one study disputed this claim. Also used as a treatment for recurrent breast cysts (Ooman, 1998). The essential fatty acids and amino acids in the seeds are reportedly good for treating mild depression. Evening primrose oil (EPO) has been used successfully with vitamin B6 therapy to treat breast pain (mastalgia). The oil is considered anticoagulant, demulcent, and a precursor of prostaglandin E (anti-inflammatory). EPO has not proven effective against multiple sclerosis (MS). Some practitioners suggest that flaxseed (omega-3 oils) and Vitamin D may better serve the MS patient as alpha-linolenic acid and Vitamin D are required for normal myelin composition.
One study showed that with women who had recurrent breast cysts, evening primrose oil treatment resulted in a slightly lower rate of recurrence as compared to placebo.
Another study suggests that EPO may reverse neurological damage in diabetic patients. Provided significantly increased serum essential fatty acids in insulin-dependent children. Also, decreased PGE2 levels.
EPO therapy may improve liver function in alcoholics and is said to decrease the use of nonsteroidal anti-inflammatory drugs in treatment for rheumatoid arthritis. Vaginal suppositories of EPO soften the cervix in preparation for labor and delivery (Senner, 2003).

Warning: In large doses may cause headache, diarrhea, indigestion, and nausea. Avoid in cases of schizophrenia and epileptogenic drugs: phenothiazines. No long-term studies during pregnancy and lactation.

Notes: Evening primrose oil is high in GLA, a naturally occurring nutrient also found in breast milk. This widely used nutritional supplement has been marketed for over thirty years.

Veterinarian/Wildlife: Seeds are fine additions to bird feeders; finches, spar-rows, and numerous other birds will be attracted to the seed-laden capsules of the plants. Omega 6 essential fatty acids from evening primrose are a constituent in Healthy Coat Skin & Coat Tabs from Doctors Foster and Smith.

Purslane

Portulacaceae (Portulaca oleracea L.)

Identification: Spreading, fleshy, succulent annual that sprawls close to the ground. Stems many branched, reddish. Leaves 1" long and thick, fleshy, smooth and shiny, ovate or teardrop shaped (spatula shaped). Small, inconspicuous, yellowish flower in leaf rosettes. Blooms June through November.

Habitat: Found nationwide, in gardens and waste ground.

Food: Purslane is a common garden plant, a volunteer alien creeper. It may be eaten right off the ground, put in salads, or chopped and added to soup. The payoff is omega-3 essential fatty acids. Native Americans ate the leaves as a raw or cooked vegetable. It was also boiled in soups and with meats. Try it chopped in salads, in salad dressing, or even in turkey stuffing. Mexicans eat purslane raw with meat and green chiles or cooked with onions, carrots, beans, and chiles. Purslane can be dried and reconstituted as a winter food.

Traditional uses: Used as a poultice and a skin lotion. The whole plant in decoction was used to treat worms. Juice of the whole plant considered a tonic and was also used to treat earaches. Purslane was an antidote to unspecified herbal toxins. Infusion of leaf stems was used to stem diarrhea. Mashed plant was applied as poultice over burns and bruises. Decoction of the whole plant was considered an antiseptic wash. Purslane was eaten to alleviate stomachache.

Modern uses: Purslane's essential fatty acids may help prevent inflammatory conditions such as heart disease, diabetes, and arthritis. Preparation of the extract is found in a few commercially available skin lotions. Ongoing clinical trial: Patients are enrolled in a clinical trial using purslane extract to treat oral lichen planus, a chronic inflammatory disease that rarely undergoes spontaneous remission. Patients with OLP have a significant increased risk of oral squamous cell (Agha-Hosseini, 2010).

Notes: Purslane is often present in commercial bags of garden manure; spread it on your garden and by midsummer, purslane. I add the succulent leaves to salads and encourage this plant to grow in my garden. It is a natural and tasty way to get omega-3 fatty acids into my diet. If you won't eat it, add it to your mulch pile. The worms will prosper!

Veterinarian/Wildlife: In Mexico this is an important fodder for wildlife and domestic animals, especially free-range chickens, providing essential fatty acids.

Red Clover

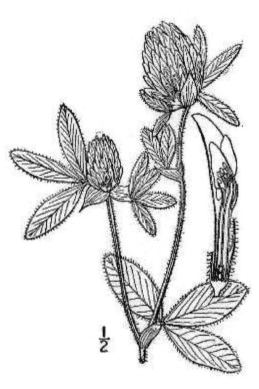

Fabaceae *(Trifolium pratense L.)*

Identification: A perennial, red clover has three leaves with a distinct V marking on each leaflet. Leaflets are fine toothed, ovate. Flowers pink to red, dome shaped or rounded in a dense terminal cluster. Grows to 12" to 18".

Habitat: Found in full sun in fields, roadsides, waste ground, along hiking trails, and abandoned railroad beds nationwide.

Medicinal part: flower and leaves.

Solvent: Boiling water.

Effects: Alterative, antispasmodic, expectorant

Traditional uses: Floral tea traditionally used as a panacea, a cure-all. Decoction or tea used as an external wash on burns, wounds, and insect bites. Pioneers claimed drinking the tea purified the blood, an enervating tonic. Tea is considered an expectorant as therapy for respiratory problems such as: asthma, cough, bronchitis, and whooping cough. Floral tea also used as an antispasmodic and mild sedative. Red clover is also used as a wash for psoriasis and eczema. Isoflavone estrogen-like compounds in clover are used to treat menopausal and postmenopausal problems.

Modern uses: A red clover isoflavone concentrate in tablet form reduced bone loss in a double-blind placebo-controlled trial with 177 women between the ages of 49 and 65 years (Adamson, Compston, Day). A smaller trial showed that red clover derivatives reduced hot flashes (van de Weijer; Barentsen). And a third study showed a 23 percent increase in arterial blood flow to the heart in women (Nestel). Red clover is still used to treat menopausal symptoms and it may improve blood flow in the heart. Standardized extracts are used, and should only be used under the supervision of a licensed health-care practitioner. The drug may increase bleeding and has other side effects.

Warning: Because of potential increased bleeding time from clover chemistry, floral teas should be used sparingly or not at all, unless supervised by a holistic health-care professional.

Red Root

Ceanothus spp.

Identification: A genus of shrubs and small trees of Rhamnaceae. There are about thirty-five species native to North America.

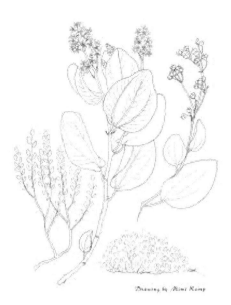

Drawing by Mimi Kamp

In California, red root grows often as small trees. In Colorado, the common species is *Ceanothus fendleri*. This type of red root is most often encountered as a scruffy, semi-thorny ground cover spreading over fairly good sized areas. The seed pods are a brilliant dark reddish color, about the same color of the tincture that is made from the roots. They are small, about half the size of a pea, and triangular. Before pods form, the branches grow small, fragrant clusters of white flowers, though in the California varieties the flowers may be lilac, pink, or purple. The stems have many sharp thorny projections and during harvesting can be painful. The exterior bark of the root is a dark to black color that, when scraped with the fingernail, will reveal a bright reddish inner bark. The more brilliant red this inner bark, the more potent the herb. The root is best harvested in the spring or fall when the reddish color is most pronounced. When most potent, the core of the root has a slight pinkish tinge. This tinge can be seen to extend throughout the whole root.

The root is very woody and should be cut when fresh into two-inch pieces. When completely dry the root is extremely hard and is very difficult to cut into smaller pieces.

Habitat: Plants of all this genus can be found on dry, sunny hillsides from coastal scrub lands to open forest clearings, from near sea level to 9,000 feet (2,700 m) in elevation. They are profusely distributed throughout the Rocky Mountains from British Columbia south through Colorado, the Cascades of Oregon and California, and the Coastal Ranges of California. The typical habitat of *Ceanothus fendleri* is pine forests from 4,900 to 9,800 ft in altitude.

Medicinal part: the root.

Solvent: Boiling water.

Effects: Astringent, Expectorant, Sedative, Antispasmodic.

Traditional uses: From a a translation of the Catawba uses of red root: "Red root is good indeed. It is a good medicine root for the mouth of a child. When the little one's mouth is sore, wash with it. The roots of red root will prove good when nipples become sore. Using the red root make it up into medicine. You will be better and the little child will be better."

Modern uses: The official root contains a large amount of prussic acid, which has been given the name "Ceanothine" and used as its active principle.

Red root is a remarkable herb, primarily for the lymph system. It helps the lymph system process waste cells very quickly and reduces the time the body suffers from colds or flu. A number of herbalists have reported that red root increases T-cell count and is a useful adjunct for immune system disorders including AIDS.

Dose and usage: Red root is beneficial for inflamed tonsils, sore throat, and enlarged lymph nodes of any location. For inflamed tonsils or sore throat, the herbal tincture should be taken in the mouth, mixed with saliva and allowed to dribble directly down the throat onto the affected areas. Recommended dosage is 30 drops of the tincture per 150 pounds of weight, three times a day for chronic conditions, up to six times a day in acute episodes.

Veterinarian/Wildlife: One of the favorite foods among deers. It makes up to 10% of the summer forage for the Arizonan mule deer.

Sageshrub

Asteraceae (Artemisia tridentata Nutt.)

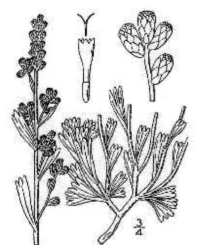

Identification: Gray, fragrant shrub to 7'. Leaves are wedge shaped, lobed (three teeth), broad at tip, tapering to the base. Yellow and brownish flowers form spreading, long, narrow clusters. Bloom in July to October. Seed is hairy achene. Also referred to as sagebrush.

Habitat: Definitive shrub in dry areas of Wyoming, Washington, Montana, Texas, New Mexico, California, Idaho, Oregon, Colorado, and elsewhere in the West.

Food: Seeds, raw or dried, are ground into flour and eaten as a survival food. Seeds have been added to liqueurs for fragrance and flavor.

Traditional uses: This powerful warrior plant is used for smudging and sweeping to rid the victim of bad airs and evil spirits. Leaves are used as a tea to treat infections or ease childbirth or as a wash for sore eyes. Leaves are soaked in water and applied as a poultice over wounds. The tea is used to treat stomachache. Tree limbs are used as switches in sweat baths. The infusion was used to treat sore throats, coughs, colds, and bronchitis. A decoction or infusion was used as a wash for sores, cuts, and pimples. The aromatic decoction of steaming herb was inhaled for respiratory ailments and headaches. The decoction was said to be internally anti-diarrheal and externally antirheumatic. This panacea drug was also drunk to relieve constipation.

Modern uses: Still very popular and important in Native American religious rituals, including smudging, sweeping, sweat lodge, and as a disinfectant. For details see the DVD Native American Medicine. Gram-positive bacteria are sensitive to the oil of A. tridentata.

Notes: Add this herb to your hot bath, hot tub, or sweat lodge for a fragrant, disinfecting, and relaxing cleanse. Often sagebrush is the only source of firewood in the desert.

Veterinarian/Wildlife: Native Americans rubbed the herb over their bodies to hide the human scent when hunting. Considered a moth and flea repellent, the decoction of the herb was applied to the wounds of domestic animals.

Sassafras

Lauraceae (Sassafras albidum [Nutt.] Nees)

Identification: A small to medium tree to 50'. Leaves mitten-shaped and irregular. Twigs and root aromatic, odor somewhat like root beer. Flowers are yellow green. Branches and twigs break easily.

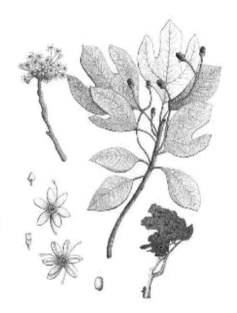

Habitat: Eastern forests and Midwestern and prairie states. Located along edges of woods, in drier, well-drained areas as a first-growth companion with oak and hickory in eastern forests.

Food: Spring leaves are dried and used as filé in gumbo and other Cajun dishes. Simply crush the dried leaves to powder and use as a spice. Spread the leaf powder on pasta, soup, cheese, and other savory dishes. For root tea, peel the root, discard the peel, and boil the pith.

Traditional uses: Extracts were used to make perfume and root beer. The root oil was used as an antiseptic until 1960, when the USDA declared it unsafe because of the content of safrole, a carcinogen. The root decoction was used in traditional healing as a drinkable tonic and blood purifier to relieve acne, syphilis, gonorrhea, arthritis, colic, menstrual pain, and upset stomach. Bark tea was used to cause sweating.

Modern uses: Sassafras has no proven effect as a medicine, and because of the toxic effects of safrole, the root tea should be taken judiciously. Small amounts of the dried leaves of spring are used as a spice. A twig chew is refreshing but overuse is not recommended. Recent evidence shows safrole, a component in sassafras oil, is added as an adulterant to the drug Ecstasy in Cambodia.

Warning: Sassafras oils, including safrole, may be carcinogenic.

Notes: When camping, you can use the twigs as a toothbrush (chew stick). Chew the end of the twig until it is bristly, then "worry" the bristles between teeth and gums. Slippery elm twigs, rich in antioxidants, also make fine chewing sticks. The flavor is refreshing and the sap is a mild sialagogue (promoting the secretion of saliva). Dried leaves make a fine tea.

Saint John's Wort

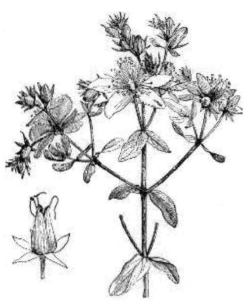

Hyperacaceae *(Hypericum perforatum L.)*

Identification: Stiff, almost woody stem, reddish and erect; may grow to 4' in height. Leaves ovate, attached at the base, and covered by glands. Hold 1.5" leaves toward the sun and you will see the glands; they appear as small perforations in the leaf. Stems bear yellow flowers with five sepals in terminal cymes (clusters). Sepals are marked with numerous glands. Blossoms have numerous stamens fused into three bundles. Cylindrical seeds are 1 to 3 mm long, black or brown, covered with small warty markings.

Habitat: Nationwide. Roadsides, waste ground, fields, prairies, stream banks, riverbanks. There are numerous garden varieties.

Traditional uses: The whole-plant decoction was used to induce abortions by promoting menstruation. Parts used included the fresh and dried flowers, buds, and leaves. Topical applications rubbed on sores may have antiviral, antibacterial, and wound-healing activity. It was considered anti-inflammatory, antibacterial, antiviral, antidiarrheal, and astringent. Traditionally used for 2,000 years, initially in Greece to drive out evil spirits. Flower infusion or flower tincture was said to calm nerves, relieve insomnia, and boost mood by dispelling lethargy, like a nervine. Internally, tea was used as a PMS treatment. Tea, standardized capsule, and tincture were used to treat sciatica, anxiety, shingles, and fibrositis. Chewed root was considered a snakebite remedy. Crushed leaves and flowers were stuffed in nose to stem nosebleed.

Modern uses: Several studies in Europe show the benefit of this herb to treat mild depression. A standardized extract of 0.3 percent hypericin, 300 milligrams three times a day, was found comparable in antidepressant effect to a drug standard of imipramine. A recent study suggests a 5 percent hyperforin extract of the plant showed a slight increase in cognitive function. Other trials suggest that the drug may combat fatigue, relieve anxiety, improve sleep, help with weight loss, and attenuate menopausal symptoms. One study showed it relieved some forms of atopic dermatitis but was no more effective than placebo for treating major depression. It may work better than fluoxetine in treating depression (M. Fava et al., 1995). A recent NIH/Duke University Medical Center study showed no difference between placebo and Saint-John's wort for treating moderate and/or severe depression (NIH/Duke University, 2012).

An external infusion of flowers and leaves is used as a cooling, astringent, wound-healing infection fighter. It is antiviral and anti-inflammatory and is said to promote healing when used externally as a poultice or wash for infections, burns, bruises, sprains, tendonitis, sprains, neuralgia, or cramps. In vitro studies show a widespread antimicrobial activity against influenza, herpes simplex I and II, retrovirus, polio virus, sindbis virus, murine cytomegalovirus, hepatitis C, and gram negative and gram positive bacteria. It appears that exposure to ultraviolet light increases its antimicrobial activity.

Saint-John's-wort is available over the counter as a dietary supplement. Check with your health practitioner for appropriate use and dosage.

Warning: Not to be used to treat severe depression or bipolar depression. Extracts when used in German trials induced side effects in 2.4 percent of the test group. Side effects included gastrointestinal irritation, restlessness, and mild allergic reactions. It appears to be synergistic with serotonin reuptake inhibitors, thereby increasing serotonin levels. Use of the supplement may lower activity of simultaneously administered drugs, including nonsedating antihistamines, oral contraceptives, certain antiretrovirals, antiepileptics, calcium channel blockers, cyclosporine, some chemotherapeutics, antibiotics, and select antifungals. Recent evidence suggests the chronic long-term use (abuse) of Saint-John's-wort is undesirable and may have negative health consequences. Purchase prepared products and only after consultation with your health-care professional.

Seneca Snakeroot

Polygalaceae *(Polygala senega)*

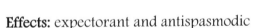

Identification: This indigenous plant has a perennial, firm, hairy, branching root, with a thick bark, and sends up several annual stems, which are erect, smooth, 8-14 in. high, occasionally tinged with red. The leaves are alternate, nearly sessile lanceolate with a sharpish point, smooth. The new, small white flowers consists of five sepals, three petals and the capsules are small, two-celled and two-valved. Found in rocky woods and on hillsides, flowering in July. The English name is Milkwort.

Habitat: Polygala is a genus of more than 500 annual and perennial herbs and shrubs of the family Polygalaceae. Most species are sub- tropical but nearly 200 are North American. P. senega, known as Mountain flax or Senega snakeroot, grows from New Brunswick to Alberta and southward to Georgia and Arkansas.

Effects: expectorant and antispasmodic

Medicinal Part: The root.

Solvents: Water, dilute alcohol.

Traditional uses: At the beginning of the eighteenth-century the Scottish physician Tennant heard from the Senega Indians of the use of Senega in cases of snake bites; and investigated its merits. He discovered that an infusion of the dried roots would actively promote salivation.

The Ojibwa call Seneca snakeroot *bi'jikiwuk'*. The name translates, literally, as "buffalo medicine". When made into medicine among the Ojibwa, Seneca snakeroot is usually combined with one to seven other herbs, the resulting combination also called *bi'jikiwuk*. Seneca snakeroot is considered to be the principal herb, without which the preparation would not be efficacious. *Bi'jikiwuk'* was the principal war medicine carried by the Ojibwa. It was said to make men strong and to be a powerful healing medicine. An Ojibwa warrior's custom was to chew it and spray it from the lips on his body and equipment. The herb was considered to be effective in counteracting negative influences directed toward a person. It was taken four times daily all throughout life and was considered to enhance and increase the vitality and personal power of the person taking it.

Dose and usage: It is useful for colds and flu, for croup, pleurisy, chronic catarrh, asthma, and coughs. It is also used as an anti-inflammatory in rheumatism and as a poultice for swellings. The root also induces sweating and is a moderately good diuretic.

<u>Slippery Elm</u>

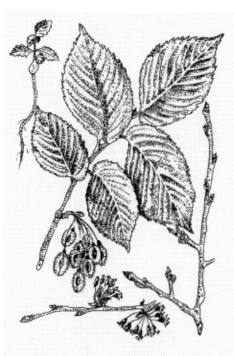

Ulmaceae (*Ulmus rubra* Muhl.)

Identification: Deciduous tree to 70' in height. Spreading branches with an open crown. Older bark rough and fissured; young branches reddish brown and downy. Leaf buds large and downy. Leaves obovate to oblong, darker green on top, rough to the touch, with a double serrated toothed margin; to 8", typically shorter. Flowers with up to nine sepals and stamens grow in dense, sessile clusters. Spinning top-shaped fruit grows to 1" long.

Habitat: North America, typically east of the Missouri River. Forests and fields.

Effects: Demulcent, emollient, expectorant, diuretic, astringent

Medicinal Part: The inner and outer bark

Solvents: Water, dilute alcohol.

Traditional uses: The inner bark in infusion was traditionally used to treat gastritis and ulcers. The bark extract from this tree acts as an antioxidant and, because it is mucilaginous and demulcent, as an emollient. Externally the extract is an excellent wound dressing, often used on burns and to treat gout, rheumatism, and arthritis. Internal uses included treating gastritis and ulcers of the stomach and duodenum. The outer bark was used to induce abortions.

Modern uses: Slippery elm is still used by holistic medicine practitioners to treat colds, sore throats, and bronchitis. The outer bark is used to make salve. The inner bark is dried and powdered, then added to water and drunk for gastric ulcers, duodenal ulcers, and colitis. It is considered antisyphilitic and antiherpetic, claims that are not yet substantially proven. The bark fraction is used in the Essiac cancer remedy, an unproven combination of slippery elm bark, sheep sorrel, burdock root, and turkey rhubarb root. These compounds may be purchased as lozenges, powder, or cut and sifted for making tea as a demulcent for respiratory irritations. See your licensed professional holistic health-care practitioner for consultation.

Dose and usage: Decoction: Mix 1 part powder to 8 parts water (mix the powder with small amount cold water initially to insure the mixing)

Usna

Parmeliaceae (*Usnea spp.*)

Identification: Parasitic epiphyte, a tree lichen, a fungus living symbiotically with an algae. There are numerous hairlike parasitic organisms hanging from conifers. Usnea is light gray-green and best identified by teasing apart the outer mycelia sheath of its skin to expose a tough white central core or cord, threadlike and supple. Other clinging lichens do not have this white central core. Also called old man's beard.

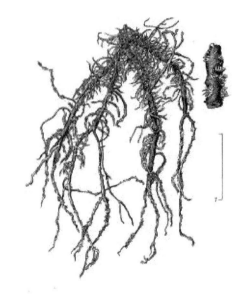

Habitat: Forests of the Pacific Northwest and in the broader north temperate climate zone of the West; worldwide in moist and damp habitats.

Medicinal Part: The whole plant.

Solvent: Water.

Effects: Carminative, Mucilaginous, Demulcent, Antiseptic.

Traditional uses: Native Americans moistened the crushed plant and applied it as a poultice over boils and wounds. In Traditional Chinese Medicine it is used to treat tuberculosis. In Europe and Asia, it was used for thousands of years as an anti-infective.

Modern uses: Commission E–approved for mouth inflammations and inflammations of the pharynx. Widely used by naturopaths to treat acute bacterial and fungal infections. Scientific studies report that the extract is effective against gram-positive bacteria (pneumococcus and streptococcus). Antiviral effects have been shown in vitro. Where available, the drug is produced in the form of lozenges. Usnea species contain antioxidants as tested in vitro.

Dose and usage: Powdered or whole it can be applied to skin infections with excellent results. Tinctured in alcohol, eaten whole, or infused as a tea, it can be taken for internal problems from tuberculosis to acute bacterial infections. As a douche it can be used to treat trichomonas and yeast infections. Herbalists generally use usnea clinically for fungus infections, acute bacterial infection, lupus, trichomonas, mastitis, varicose and tropic ulcers, second- and third-degree burns, plastic surgery, athlete's foot, ringworm, urinary tract infections, colds, flu, bronchitis, pleurisy, pneumonia, tuberculosis, sinus infections, staphylococcus, dysentery, and streptococcus.

Notes: Campers used the lichen as stuffing material for mattresses, pillows, as a soft bedding under sleeping bag. Moerman reports that the Nitinaht women used usnea as sanitary napkins and as diaper material for babies (Moerman, 1998).

Valerian

Valerianaceae (Valeriana sitchensis Bong.; V. officinalis L.)

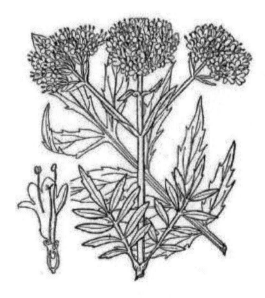

Identification: Perennial to 24", sometimes taller. Leaves opposite, staggered up the stem, often with several basal leaves. Terminal cluster of white- to cream-colored odiferous flowers; petals are feathery. Blooms April to July.

Habitat: Montane plant, typically found on north-facing slopes. Plentiful in alpine meadows and along trails in the Olympics, Cascades, North Cascades, Mount Rainier, and Mount Baker, especially along Heliotrope Trail toward the climbers' route.

Medicinal Part: The root.

Solvent: Water.

Effects: Antispasmodic, Calmative, Stimulating Tonic, Nervine.

Traditional uses: Stress-reducing, tension-relieving mild sedative for insomniacs. V. sitchensis roots were decocted in water to treat pain, colds, and diarrhea. A poultice of the root was used to treat cuts, wounds, bruises, and inflammation.

Modern uses: A few people still use V. sitchensis in the traditional way. Aqueous extract of V. officinalis root in a doubleblind study had significant relaxing effect on poor or irregular sleepers, smokers. Sometimes combined with hops (Humulus lupulus) and skullcap (Scutellaria lateriflora). Valerian is used by herbalists today as a nerve tonic. Is best combined with Skull cap (Scutellaria), Blue vervain (Verbena hastata), and Mistletoe (Viscum album), Gentian (Gentiana lutea) and Peppermint (Mentha piperita) increase the promptness of its action, which is more effective than when combined with bromide. The effect of valerian on gamma amino butyric acid (GABA) may reduce blood pressure and help mild depression. This chemical is also found in evening primrose seeds and several varieties of tomatoes.

Watercress

Brassicaceae (Nasturtium officinale L.)

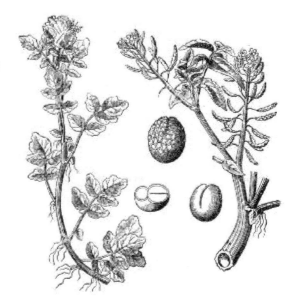

Identification: Water-loving plant that grows in floating mats that root beneath the water and rise as much as 14" above. Grooved stem is tough, fibrous when mature. Leaves alternate, ovate, with paired and lobed leaflets. Each leaflet broader toward the base and about ¾" wide, but variable in width, with terminal lobe. White flower, ¼" wide, with four petals. Blooms in May and sporadically through summer and may be available year-round if warmer weather persists.

Habitat: Nationwide. Temperate areas; in or near seeps and springs, along the margins of slow-moving, muck-bottomed streams and creeks.

Medicinal Parts: Leaves, root.

Solvent: Water.

Effects: Tonic, Stimulant, Blood purifying.

Food: Watercress is from the mustard family, and its taste is spicy and pungent. Harvest watercress from a clean water source, then cook it. That's right—trust only your backyard if you plan to eat this food raw. You may pull watercress out by its roots and replant it in your garden. Keep it wet and it will reward you with peppery leaves. It is one of the main ingredients in V8 vegetable juice. Watercress is great in Italian dishes: Try it mixed half and half with spinach in spinach lasagna.

Traditional uses: The pharmaceutical record all the way back to Hippocrates describes watercress as a heart tonic, stimulating expectorant, and digestive. It is good for coughs, colds, and bronchitis and it relieves gas. As a diuretic it releases fluid retention and cleanses the kidneys and bladder. Mexicans revere this plant as a spring tonic. It is dampened and then grilled over charcoal.

Modern uses: Watercress is a good source of vitamins, minerals, and isothiocyanate. Watercress in 8 ounces of V8 cocktail juice provides two servings of vegetables. The latter may provide protection from cancer and is Commission E–approved to treat coughs and bronchitis.

Notes: Watercress, often found growing wild in questionable water sources, should be relocated to your garden. Keep it well watered and it will cleanse itself.

Veterinarian/Wildlife: Mats of watercress are habitats for snails, insect larvae, and frogs. These creatures attract fish. Should you find a mat on your favorite trout stream, approach cautiously and expect to be surprised.

White Poplar

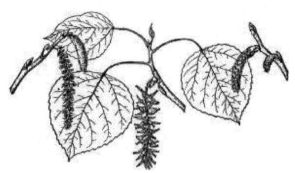

Salicaceae (Populus spp.: P. balsamifera L.; P. tremuloides Michx.; P. deltoides Bartr. ex Marsh)

Identification: Many poplars have ovate leaves on long petioles that provide a quaking effect when the wind blows. Flowers are drooping catkins. Cottonwood (P. deltoides) when mature has thick, furrowed bark. Aspen (P. tremuloides) is distinctive with its greenish-white bark and quaking leaves. Balsam poplar (P. balsamifera) has broad heart-shaped leaves, 6" to 10", edged with fine teeth; slightly flattened to rounded leaf stalks. New-growth end buds of balsams are sticky (resinous) and aromatic. The young balsam poplar's bark is gray green and smooth; the mature tree has dark, grooved bark.

Habitat: Wide distribution in United States. Requires ample water. Balsam poplar is found in the northern tier of states and throughout southern and central Canada. Cottonwoods reside typically in low, wet areas. Aspens are found in stands on mountain slopes, in mountain meadows, and along wild rivers.

Medicinal Parts: Leaves, bark, buds.

Solvent: Boiling water (soak buds in alcohol, then boiling water will expel their properties).

Effects: Tonic, Diuretic, Stimulant, Febrifuge.

Food: Balsam poplar cambium (inner bark) is eaten raw. The cambium was boiled, dried, pounded to flour, and mixed with corn flour (masa) and/or wheat flour to make bread. Shoots, leaf buds, and catkins taste best when simmered in water. The vitamin C content is high.

Traditional uses: Native Americans considered balsam poplar a panacea: The inner bark decoction was used as a tonic, a treatment for colds, and a system cleanser after acute infections. The bark maceration and decoction was used as a wash for rheumatism. Pioneers gathered the reddish resin covering new-growth leaf buds and dissolved and thinned the resin in an alcohol solvent. The resulting salve was applied to seal and heal wounds and relieve inflammations.

Modern uses: Bark, leaves, and leaf buds are used in modern therapies. Leaf bud extract is Commission E–approved to treat hemorrhoids, wounds, and burns. The leaf-bud extract is healing, antibacterial, and antiphlogistic (relieves inflammation). Salicin from the bark and leaves is analgesic (it's considered a precursor of aspirin, the synthetic of which was modeled after the natural drug). The bark and leaves are considered antispasmodic and are used to treat arthritis, rheumatism, and pain and urinary complaints due to prostate hypertrophy. The bitter tonic effect and alterative effect may make it helpful in treating anorexia.

Warning: Do not use poplar if you are allergic to aspirin or other salicylates.

Notes: Poplar is not a particularly good firewood. Although poplar tree sap may be tapped, its sugar content is low, and too much boiling is required to sweeten the brew.

Veterinarian/Wildlife: Young trees, leaf buds, and shoots are browsed on by deer, moose, and rodents. Dead and dying poplars are a favorite place to find oyster mushrooms.

<u>Willow</u>

Salicaceae (Salix spp.: S. alba L.; S. nigra Marsh)

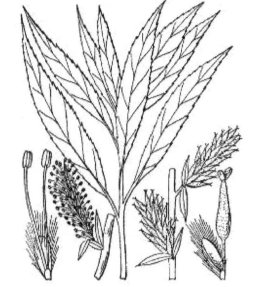

Identification: Tree or shrub from 10' to over 100' with lancelike fine-toothed leaves; yellow male flowers and green female flowers in the form of densely blossomed catkins. White willow (S. alba), sometimes called weeping willow, has drooping branches. Black willow (S. nigra) is erect, large with shedding branches. Both prefer wet ground and are considered dirty trees in that they constantly shed branches, flowers, and leaves.

Habitat: Nationwide north to the Arctic. Marshy areas, mountain streams, thickets, lakeshores, along streams and rivers.

Medicinal Part: The bark.

Solvent: Boiling water.

Effects: Aphrodisiac, Tonic, Astringent, Detergent.

Traditional uses: Native Americans used the bark of twigs and new growth in decoction to treat tendonitis, arthritis, headaches, and bursitis. An infusion of the stem and leaves releases salicin, the natural chemical model for synthetic aspirin. Aspirin may help prevent acute infections, cancer, strokes, and heart attacks. It may help boost immunity, but it does have numerous side effects and may aggravate ulcers and cause intestinal bleeding.

Modern uses: The extraction, although infrequently used from the tree, is Commission E–approved for treating pain and rheumatism. Not to be used by people allergic to salicyclates. **Warning:** Much double-blind, placebo-controlled, double-crossover research has been done on aspirin but not on salicin from willow extraction. Keep in mind that the infusion or decoction of willow contains much more than salicin. Recent evidence shows that willow can concentrate cadmium, a toxic metal, in its tissue. All species of willow are known to concentrate this metal when it is available in the soil. I prefer using aspirin for its therapeutic effects.

Notes: Do not garden under or too near a willow. Willow rootlets travel near the surface and suck water and nutrients from the soil. This can distress nearby garden plants. When a willow dies, be aware that the widespread root system has drained the soil of nutrients. Rebuild the soil before you replant the area.

Witch Hazel

Hamamelidaceae *(Hamamelis virginiana L.)*

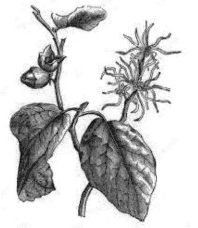

Identification: Deciduous small bushy tree or shrub to 10' in height, occasionally much taller. Bark thin, brown on the outside, red on the inside. Younger branches haired and yellow brown. Leaves alternate, blunt, indented, with rough margins. Five to seven yellow, short-stemmed flowers appear in clusters before leaves emerge, a golden appearance. Flowers grow from the axils of leaf buds. Petals are bright, long, narrow, linear, and roll to a spiral in the bud. Fruit capsule oddly shaped, woody, oval, about ¾" long.

Habitat: Typically east of the Mississippi River. Coastal forests. I find it growing along trails, specifically Grand Mere State Park, Stevensville, Michigan.

Medicinal Part: The bark and concrete juice.

Solvent: Boiling water and alcohol.

Effects: Stimulant, Expectorant, Diuretic, Antiseptic, Disinfectant.

Traditional uses: Witch hazel was used by the Cherokee, Chippewa, Iroquois, Mohegan, Menominee, and Potawatomi peoples living in the range of the plant east of the Mississippi. They used the leaf tea externally to treat muscle aches, athlete's foot, wounds, burns, and various skin afflictions. Tea was consumed for coughs, asthma, colds, sore throats, dysentery, and diarrhea. Twigs and inner bark are still used in infusion to treat colds, pain, sores, fevers, sore throat, and tuberculosis. An infusion of twigs was used to treat dysentery and diarrhea. A decoction of new-growth tips and shoots from the base of the plant was used as a blood purifier or spring tonic. Young end tips were used in decoction to treat colds and coughs. Root and twig decoctions were considered a cure-all for just about any ailment: bruises, edema, cholera, and arthritis.

Modern uses: Twigs are steam-distilled to yield witch hazel water, to which 14 percent alcohol is added to form witch hazel extract. This very old medicinal remedy continues to be sold today as an over-the-counter (OTC) medicine. It is one of the few nonprescription "drugs" that has received FDA approval as an OTC astringent, skin protectant, and analgesic. It has been sold for these uses for more than 200 years. Modern science has shown that the extract has antiviral properties as well. Witch hazel water is distilled from the leaves and twigs and used as an eyewash and to treat hemorrhoids, colitis, varicose veins, sore muscles, bruises, and sprains. Tannins derived from distilling the active compound are used to treat local skin irritations and inflammations, including eczema. Distilled witch hazel water contains no tannins but is still astringent and is used as a gargle for sore throat and sore gums.

Notes: Twigs of witch hazel have traditionally been used to fashion divining rods for the art of dowsing, which is the practice of seeking locations where groundwater exists before digging or drilling a water well. Early Americans called this practice "water witching," because witch hazel was one of the branches of choice, although willow and peach tree branches were sometimes employed instead.

A flexible Y- or L-shaped twig was held in front of a person, while the person moved slowly across the area where ground¬water was being sought. If the twig inclined downward or twitched, then that movement was thought to indicate the presence of water below the surface.

Wormwood

Asteraceae *(Artemisia campestris L. subsp. caudata* [Michx.] H.M. Hall & Clem.*)*

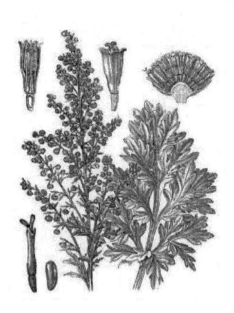

Identification: Artemisia species comprise numerous plants found worldwide. A. campestris is not aromatic, unlike many other artemisias. It is a biennial, a second-year flowering plant or a shortlived perennial. First-year leaves are a basal rosette, each leaf up to 4" long and 3" wide. Leaves are deeply divided with narrow, linear lobes; color is grayish blue. Upper mature (second-year) leaves have a green undersurface and whitish-green top. On the mature plant, leaves get smaller and more deeply cut or linear toward the top of the plant. Leaves are hairy at first and become smooth as they mature. Stems are branched, light green to red in color. Young stem ends are matte with fine hairs. The cobweblike hairs disappear as the stem grows. Also known as dune wormwood or field sagewort. Many species of wormwood, also known as mugwort, are called "sage." This is a misnomer as they are not related to the sage family and cannot be used interchangeably.

Habitat: In Michigan, frequently found in Great Lakes dunes area. Widely dispersed, however, from coast to coast and south to Texas and north into Canada. Away from dunes, search on dry roadsides, sides of hills, and other dry, sandy areas.

Medicinal Parts: The tops and leaves.

Solvents: Diluted alcohol, water (partially).

Effects: Tonic, Stomachic, Stimulant, Febrifuge, Anthelmintic, Narcotic.

Food: Not edible. The leaves of Artemisia species are often made into bitter teas to treat indigestion. Absinthe from other Artemisia species is used to flavor vermouth and other spirits, to include the cordial absinthe.

Traditional uses: Tewa nation people chewed and swallowed juice to relieve gas and upset stomach. Leaf infusion also used to treat fever and chills (see Moerman, p. 93).
The herb has traditionally been used as a smudging agent. The green plant is cut and gathered together in a bundle and wrapped with small string and allowed to dry. The end is lit and used as a "smudge wand" in ceremonial smudging. The plant is also used, dry or moistened, in the sweat lodge. The plant is placed on the hot stones in the center of the lodge and the resulting vapor inhaled.
Numerous people and holistic practitioners have used the plant as medicine for thousands of years, particularly popular in Europe and China.

Modern uses: Thujone and artemisinin are anthelmintic, that is, they kill intestinal worms (including the malaria falciparum) and other parasites. In Europe wormwood (Artemisia) is used as a stomach bitters and digestive (an after-dinner drink, such as vermouth or absinthe, relieves indigestion). Artimisinin, a synthetic derivative from sweet wormwood (Artemisia annua) is used to control malaria and other parasites. Tu Youyou, who discovered this use, was awarded the Nobel Prize in 2015. A recent clinical trial showed artimisin 97 percent effective against noncomplicated cases of malaria (see ncbi.nlm.nih.gov/pmc/articles/PMC1887535).

Dose and usage: A rounded teaspoon of the dried plant in a cup of hot water, allowed to steep for fifteen minutes, is useful to promote sweating in feverish states or to increase scanty menstruation.

Wormwood tea, though bitter, is a good remedy for stomach indigestion. It has also been traditionally used, as its name suggests, in cases of intestinal worms. Michael Moore suggests two cups a day for at least two weeks, making sure its use is constant.

Warning: Thujone is a GABA antagonist—in large amounts it blocks gamma amino butyric acid, which can lead to seizures and even death. Artemisia chemistry is toxic in large enough dose, and the amount of Artemisia extract used in alcoholic drinks is government controlled.

Veterinarian/Wildlife: Wormwood extracts are used to treat worm infestations in domestic animals. There may be benefits for using Artemisia as a companion plant among vegetable and flowers. It is an attractive and unusual houseplant and garden plant.

Yarrow

Asteraceae *(Achillea millefolium L.)*

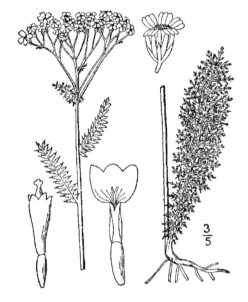

Identification: Spreading perennial with soft feather-like leaves to 3' to 4' in height. Fragrant. White flowers in flat clusters, flowers have five petal-like rays.

Habitat: Broadly distributed along roadsides, fields, yards, gardens, mountain slopes, streams, edges of woods nationwide—especially prevalent in montane areas.

Medicinal Part: The herb. Though some people prepare only the flowers as medicine, I commonly use the whole plant but leave the root. The root may be used with effectiveness but I prefer to leave it so that it can continue to produce new plants each year.

Solvents: Water, alcohol.

Effects: Astringent, Alterative, Diuretic, Tonic.

Traditional uses: Traditionally the tea made from the aerial parts (leaves and flowers) is said to increase perspiration and reduce inflammation; used both externally and internally.

In China, the tea is taken to protect against thrombosis after stroke or heart attack and is used over wounds and for hemorrhoids, inflamed eyes, nosebleeds, and ulcers. Can be combined with elderberry flowers and/or berries.

Native American uses: Yarrow is ranked as one of the most important herbs used by Native Americans.

Whole plant (aerial parts) infused and used to treat acute infections: colds, fever, flu, and as a diuretic.

Whole plant infusion is used to control coughing. Wash (infusion) of the whole plant is also used for bites, stings, snakebites.

Root decoction may be used as a wash for pimples.

Leaves are infused and consumed as tea to induce sleep, as an antidiarrheic, and to reduce fever (febrifuge).

The leaf infusion is also a poison ivy treatment.

The leaves dried, crushed, and snorted are snuff for headaches, placed in the nasal cavities they also stop nose-bleedings.

Fresh or dry leaves are used as a poultice over wounds, or as a fomentation or poultice over breast (nipple) abscesses.

Bella Coola people chewed leaves and applied them as a poultice to treat burns and boils, used leaves and flowers in decoction for headaches or for chest pains, and poultice of flowers (masticated) to reduce edema.

Finally, leaves mixed with animal fat may be used used as a poultice on the chest and back to treat bronchitis.

Modern uses: Commission E–approved to treat loss of appetite, liver and gallbladder complaints, dyspepsia, and lower abdominal pains.

In Europe the entire plant used as an antispasmodic, emmenagogue, tonic, carminative, digestive aid, and for wound healing. Infusion of the aerial parts is used as a carminative, digestive aid, tonic, and emmenagogue.

Wound healing is facilitated by an infusion in distilled water and application as a wash to the wound site.

A 70 percent alcohol extract of yarrow lowered blood lipids (PDR, 2000, p. 918). Yarrow may lower blood pressure slightly, and could strengthen the effects of prescription drugs taken to lower blood pressure (University of Maryland).

Dose and usage: Prepared as a hot tea, yarrow will stimulate perspiration. I have found the tincture useful for settling the stomach, though it is more effective in combination with other herbs such as betony and poleo mint. The herb is traditionally used to aid the body in diseases where fevers are present. It lowers the blood pressure, though marginally. I have found it effective used in conjunction with passion flower for this purpose. It stimulates digestion and tones the stomach. As such it is useful in cases of hiatal hernia where the stomach has lost tone and is protruding up through the esophagus or a tear in the muscle wall. The fresh leaves are an excellent remedy for bleeding; placed on moderate sized to small cuts they readily stimulate clotting. The tea or tincture is also excellent for decreasing menstruation during a particularly strong flow—use a full dropper of tincture every three hours.

Warning: Drinking the tea and applying the herb has induced photosensitivity, sensitivity to light. The tea may also contain a small amount of thujone, a carcinogen and liver toxin. As with all plants, allergic reactions are possible.

Notes: Yarrow is used to flavor gin and other liquors. The herb should be in everyone's garden. Yarrow is a "secret" ingredient in fine beers. The bitter tea is a good digestive and anti-inflammatory that may protect you from infection. Use it when you have been exposed to infective organisms or infected individuals. I use lard for oil extractions from this herb, because lard penetrates deeper than olive oil and other plant-based oils.

Veterinarian/Wildlife: Leaves and stems can be smudged as a mosquito repellent. Whole aerial parts may be used to preserve fish by stuffing it in the cleaned body cavity.

Yellow Dock

Rumex crispus

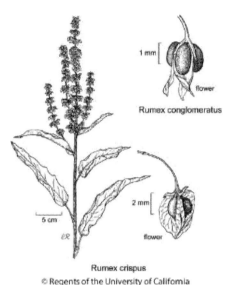

Rumex conglomeratus

Rumex crispus
© Regents of the University of California

Identification: The leaves of the yellow dock are curly-edged, a foot in length, and alternate along the stem. The plant turns a striking rust-red in the fall; during the winter the dead stalks and heavy seed panicles at the top of the two-to-three-foot stem are readily recognizable. The root is shaped something like a carrot and is reddish brown outside, yellowish to orange inside. The darker the yellow of the root the stronger the medicinal qualities of the plant. The compounds making the root yellow are the primary medicinal substances of the plant and therefore are more present the more yellow the root. Plants growing in water are not useful for medicinal purposes, therefore, gathering should take place in drier embankments and open meadows.

Habitat: Nationwide, fringes of yards, streamsides, vacant lots, roadsides, wherever you stumble along.

Taste: The yellowish spindle-shaped root has scarcely any odour, but has astringent, bitter taste.

Medicinal Part: The root.

Solvents: Water, alcohol.

Effects: Alterative, Astringent, Laxative, Antiscorbutic, Tonic.

Traditional uses: Most Native American tribes mashed the root and applied it to the skin to treat arthritis. Cherokee used the root juice for treating diarrhea. One unusual use was rubbing the throat with a crushed leaf to treat sore throat. Cooked seeds were eaten to stem diarrhea. Dried and powdered root used to stop bleeding (styptic). Pioneers considered the plant an excellent blood purifier, a spring tonic for whatever ails you.

Modern uses: Naturopaths simmer the sliced root and administer the broth to pregnant women as a source of iron, without the resulting constipation from taking elemental iron supplements. The bitter taste of the herb (root and leaves) stimulates digestion: increases hydrochloric acid secretion, increases peristalsis, and improves secretion of other digestive enzymes. Whole plant in decoction said to cleanse toxins from body and may have a laxative effect because of inherent tannins and anthraquinones (fights constipation). Considered a tonic and laxative (PDR, fourth edition, 2000).

Reported to help improve chronic skin problems. Bitter taste stimulates liver activity (blood purifier) and may help cleanse the liver, thereby relieving related skin manifestations. Sometimes combined with dandelion root to treat skin problems.

Warning: Restrict the amount of dock leaves you eat because of the high tannin content and oxalic acid content. These chemicals may be harmful to the kidneys and may negatively affect bone density when eaten in excess.

Food: Young leaves may be steamed, sautéed, or stir-fried. Be judicious; leaves may be bitter. Try steaming the herbs, then frying them in olive oil. Inner pulp of flowering stem is eaten after cooking. Squeeze pulp from skin to reduce bitterness. Seeds may be gathered and eaten.

Yew

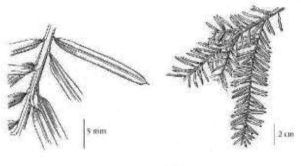
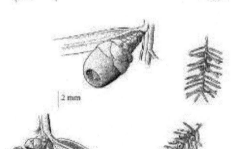

Taxus brevifolia

Rhamnaceae *(Taxus brevifolia)*

Identification: Evergreen shrub to scanty small tree to 50' in height. Bark papery, reddish-purple to red brown. Drooping branches. Flat leaves (needles), in opposite rows. Flowers are small cones. Fruit scarlet, berrylike, with fleshy cup around a single seed.

Habitat: Northern California, Oregon, and Washington through Idaho and Montana north to British Columbia and Alberta. Foothills Pacific Coast Range, moist, shady sites.

Food: According to Moerman (Native American Ethnobotany), the Karok and Mendocino tribes ate the red, ripe fruit. But the seed and all other parts of the plant are toxic. Avoid eating this plant.

Traditional uses: Native Americans used the wet needles of American yew (T. brevifolia) as a poultice over wounds. The needles were considered a panacea, a powerful tonic, and were boiled and used over injuries to alleviate pain. Bark decoctions were used to treat stomachache.

Traditionally, women of the Okanagan tribe and other northwestern coastal tribes ate yew berries as a form of contraception. The Quinault people prepared the bark as a decoction and drank it in very small doses to relieve arthritis, tuberculosis, and kidney disease. The Cowlitz Indians made a poultice of the needles and applied it topically to wounds. The leaves are not taken internally, however, as they are poisonous.

Modern uses: The toxic drug taxine (paclitaxel) from American yew is used to treat cancer. It prevents cell multiplication and may prove an effective therapy for leukemia and for cancer of the cervix, ovary, and breast. Clinical trials continue with the drug.

Warning: Both species can induce abortion. **All parts of the plant are toxic.** Unless guided by an expert, avoid eating any part of this plant.

Notes: Many North American tribes considered yew a sacred tree representing protection, strength, and manhood. The wood was used for spirit poles, shaman's rattles, drum frames, and other devotional objects. Even in Europe, the yew has long been considered sacred. For the Celts, the European species of yew, T. baccata, was one of nine sacred woods, which they burned in ritual fires.

Yucca

Agavaceae (*Yucca* spp.: *Y. filamentosa* L.; *Y. glauca* Nutt.; *Y. baccata* Torr.)

Identification: Medium to large perennials (2' to 20') with robust, ever-expanding rootstocks, often growing in clumps and colonies. Leaves swordlike, radiating out from basal rosettes, waxy (shiny) green; long, tough, and fibrous. Flowers white or cream colored; cup, bell, or bowl shaped; borne on tall woody spikes extending well above leaves. Typically flowers from May through July. Also known as Adam's needle, Spanish bayonet, or Joshua tree.

Habitat: Upland prairies, high plains, sandy blowouts, California coastal hillsides, deserts.

Food: The white flowers are edible: fold them fresh into frittatas or omelets. Garnish a plate with them. Shred them onto salads. The fruits of these plants are also edible, a few species more edible than others. Y. baccata has large succulent fruits that are bland but rich with health-protecting flavonoids.

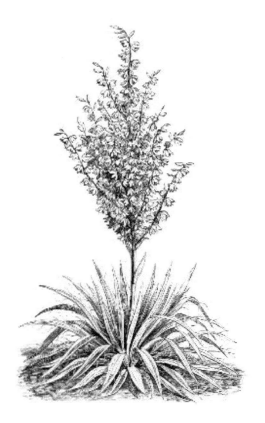

Traditional uses: Folklore claims that the root decoction will restore hair. The infusion of the smashed root was taken internally to relieve headache. Yucca root extract is a surfactant or wetting agent, capable of popping the cell membranes of microorganisms. It is therefore a useful, natural soap. Yucca root water decoction is still used to wash hair and kill lice. The root water decoction was drunk to treat arthritis (phytosterols), a potentially risky proposition with so little scientific study of the plant having been performed. See the video Little Medicine: The Wisdom to Avoid Big Medicine (appendix D). Y. filamentosa root, with its steroid saponins, has been decocted and used to treat gallbladder and liver problems. A water extraction of smashed leaves was used to quell vomiting, and root water infusion used as a laxative. The root is a male warrior plant and used in smudging rituals to rid the body of bad airs and bad spirits. The root of Y. baccata was taken to ease childbirth; this author surmises that the bitter saponins stimulated contractions.

Modern uses: In Europe leaves ground and dried and extracts of the plant are available for medicinal use. The root and leaf extraction (steroid saponins) of Adam's needle (Y. filamentosa) are still used for liver and gallbladder complaints. The side effects of too much steroid saponin intake are stomach upset and nausea. These uses are scientifically unconfirmed. Saponins in the plant lyse (kill, rupture cellular wall) bacteria and produce suds—still used as a shampoo in Native American rituals.

Zizia Aurea

Zizia Aurea (Apiaceae)

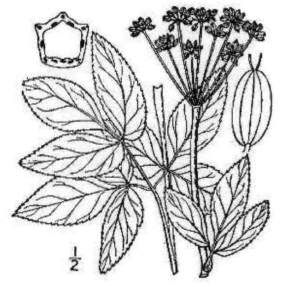

Identification: The Golden Zizia, or Golden Alexander, is an upright, native, perennial forb growing to 1 – 2 feet in height. The leaves are up to 8 centimeters long and 5 centimeters across, have finely serrated margins, generally lanceolate or ovate in shape and the larger leaves usually have 1 or 2 sharp lobes. Lower (basal) leaves are twice or three times compound with long petioles, while the upper leaves are once compound with short petioles. Golden Alexanders is most noteworthy for its attractive bright yellow flower which occurs from May – June. The flower is less than .3 centimeters long. Each flower has 5 sepals, 5 petals and 5 stamens. A cluster of flowers gathers into an 8-centimeter long flat-topped flower head, the middle flower of each compound umbel being stalk less.

Flowers give way to 3 – 4 millimeter long, oblong, green fruit capsules. The leaves as well as the fruit slowly turn light purple in the autumn.

Habitat: Widely distributed from Quebec to Saskatoon, and south to Florida and Texas. Habitats include moist black soil prairies, openings in moist to mesic woodlands, savannas, thickets, limestone glades and bluffs, power line clearings in woodland areas, and abandoned fields.

Food: The flowers can be used in salads, and the green stems can be cooked much like broccoli.

Medicinal parts: Flowers, leaves, and root.

Solvents: water

Effects: febrifuge, anesthetic

Traditional uses: Native Americans used the pulverized root to treat sharp pains; a tea was made from the leaves and flowers to treat ""female disorders""; poulticed root were used on inflammations and sores.

Dose and usage: A tea made from the root is febrifuge.

Conclusion

I hope you have enjoyed reading this book as much as I've enjoyed writing it, and I hope it will accompany you in your ongoing journey to the discovery of Native American herbs and their medicinal uses.

If you found this book useful and are feeling generous, please take the time to leave a short review on Amazon so that other may enjoy this guide as well.

I leave you with good wishes and hopefully a better knowledge of the plants around us and their amazing powers.

• The Native American Herbalist's Bible 3 •

• The Lost Book of Herbal Remedies •

The Ultimate Herbal Dispensatory to Discover the Secrets and Forgotten Practices of Native American Herbal Medicine

Linda Osceola Naranjo

Introduction

We live in a country where the cure for virtually any disease and ailment is within our grasp. In our forests, meadows, plains, and gardens grow small, seemingly insignificant flowers and herbs, plants that we don't look twice at, and trees of which we don't even bother to learn the name. Yet, they are the key to a better, healthier, and more sustainable way of life.

Our forefathers, more attuned with nature that we could ever imagine to be, understood that and took carefully and sparingly the gifts that Nature offered to heal themselves and grow stronger. We have lost that knowledge. Only starting from the 1970s, a renewed interest in botanic medicine has uncovered the depth of the Native American knowledge of plants and their healing powers. The research has not only helped herbalists, but physicians and scientist as well that re-discovered substances that the Native Americans people knew about for hundreds of years.

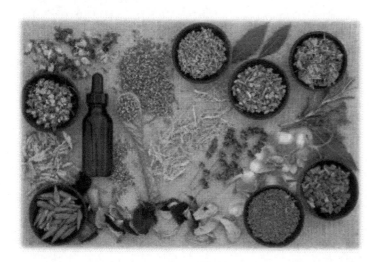

The mountains, I become a part of it...
The herbs, the fir tree, I become a part of it.
The morning mists, the clouds, the gathering waters,
I become a part of it.
The wilderness, the dew drops, the pollen...
I become a part of it.

Navajo Chant

You don't need to put at risk the delicate natural balance of your body by taking drugs and medications, if an easily available natural solution is just outside your door. Harvest carefully or grow your own herbs, learn to know your body and what works best for you, communicate with the nature surrounding you, and you will in a small way bring back a culture that for too long as been treated as inferior.

This book will teach how to find and treat the herbs the way the native American tribes did: from the forest to your herbalist table, but you will have to find your way to listen to your body and the plants around you.

To aid you in your holistic journey, we have decided to divide the book in three volumes. The first volume offers you a full theoretical approach to Native American medicine and the herbal medicines methods and preparations. The second volume is a complete encyclopedia of all the most relevant herbs used in traditional Native American medicine, complete with modern examples, doses, and where to find them, making it a very effective field guide. This third volume is a "recipe book" of sorts: it offers easy herbal solutions to the most common diseases a budding naturopath can encounter. It is meant as a jumping point to find your own way to treat yourself and your fellow man and will come in handy even to the most experienced herbalist.

Please keep in mind that, because herbs were the very first medicines, they can be very powerful. Do not gather herbs from the wild unless you know what you are doing. And please, grow your own herbs whenever possible; native herbs are becoming increasingly rare, and many are threatened with extinction.

Choosing the right herbs and herbal combinations for your health needs is most important for you. Follow three easy steps to identify and satisfy your herbal and nutritional needs:
1. Identify the injury or disorder that is affecting you.
2. Identify the areas of your health status and specific needs that require additional support.
3. Choose the most appropriate treatment program from this book that fits your needs. This should include herbs, enzymes, vitamins, minerals, and phytochemicals.

As always, if you are pregnant or nursing, if you suffer from a chronic condition such as heart disease or diabetes, or if you are currently taking medications of any kind, please consult with your physician or a well-trained herbal specialist before self-treating. Herbs and other supplements can alter the way your body utilizes other medicines. They can sometimes improve the efficacy of medicines and, at other times, interfere with the absorption or action of a particular drug.

If you have any questions about the appropriateness of any treatment, seek the services of a well-trained health-care professional. This book and the formulas contained herein are not intended to replace the services of a well-trained health-care professional.

Abscess and Gingivitis

An abscess is a local accumulation of pus. It can occur almost anywhere on or in the body, but it most frequently occurs on the skin and on the gums of the mouth. Abscesses can be very tender and painful and are marked by inflammation, swelling, heat, redness, and often fever. Abscesses are caused by an infection, so it is often treated with antibiotics. But herbs are an effective and safe alternative, without the side effects of antibiotics.

Relevant tissue states: heat (inflammation), dampness, laxity
Relevant herbal actions: anti-inflammatory, antimicrobial, astringent, vulnerary

Herbal Allies

- Barberries
- Calendula flower
- Chamomile flower
- Echinacea
- Goldenrod leaf and flower
- Licorice root
- Meadowsweet flower
- Oregon grape root
- Plantain leaf
- Rose
- Sage leaf
- Self-heal leaf and flower
- Thyme leaf
- Uva-ursi leaf
- White Oak
- Yarrow leaf and flower
- Yerba Mansa

It can be very painful to have an abscess—a fluid-filled blister or infection—in the mouth. Gingivitis is an inflammation of the gums that can lead to loose teeth. Resist the urge to poke and prod at the gums too much—if you make them bleed, bacteria can move deeper. Treat your gums gently! Antimicrobial, astringent, anti-inflammatory, and wound-healing herbs fight infection and restore healthy tissue.

HERBAL MOUTHWASH

Makes 8 fluid ounces (16 to 20 swishes)

While saltwater works well on its own, adding herbs makes it much more effective. Adjust the amounts of each herb according to taste. Swish with ¼ to ½ fluid ounce of mouthwash after brushing, and swish well, getting between the teeth and throughout the mouth, for 2 to 5 minutes.

4 fluid ounces water
1 teaspoon sea salt
1 fluid ounce tincture of uva-ursi
1 fluid ounce tincture of yarrow

½ fluid ounce tincture of calendula
½ fluid ounce tincture of plantain
½ fluid ounce tincture of self-heal
¼ fluid ounce tincture of licorice
¼ fluid ounce tincture of meadowsweet

1. In a jar with a lid, combine all the ingredients. Cover the jar, label it, and shake well. This is shelf stable.
2. Use this mouthwash every time you brush—twice a day is best.

SKIN~ABSCESS~FIGHTING TEA

30 drops echinacea tincture (See Part One for directions for tinctures.)
60 drops yerba mansa tincture
1 cup warm water

1. Combine all the ingredients.
2. Take up to five times per day to stimulate the immune system and help eliminate the infection.

TOPICAL WASH FOR ABSCESSES AND GINGIVITIS

1 to 2 teaspoons barberries
1 tablespoon white oak bark
1 teaspoon echinacea root
1 teaspoon granulated Oregon grape root
2 cups boiling water

1. Combine the herbs in a glass container.
2. Pour the boiling water over the herbs and soak for 3 to 4 hours; strain.
3. Use three times a day as a wash. If you are using this tea to treat a gum abscess, be sure to swish the liquid around in your mouth for several minutes before spitting it out.

Acne

Acne is an inflammatory skin condition that commonly affects adolescents (because of increased glandular activity during the teen years). Acne occurs when the sebaceous glands, which are located just beneath the skin, become inflamed. These glands secrete an oil called sebum, which acts to lubricate the skin. Acne results when the pores of the skin become clogged by the sebum. Acne can occur any time in life and may be due to allergies, high-sugar or high-fat diets, heredity, the use of oral contraceptives and other drugs (such as cortisone), hormone changes, and stress.

Relevant tissue states: heat (inflammation), dampness (oily)
Relevant herbal actions: anti-inflammatory, antimicrobial, astringent, circulatory stimulant, liver stimulant, lymphatic

Herbal Allies

- Burdock
- Calendula flower
- Chamomile flower
- Dandelion root
- Echinacea
- Elder
- Ginger root
- *Gingko Biloba*
- Ginseng
- Licorice
- Milk thistle seed
- Rose
- Sage leaf
- Self-heal leaf and flower
- St. John's wort leaf and flower
- Thyme leaf
- Yarrow leaf and flower
- White Willow Bark

To cope with chronic skin problems, it's important to treat the issue from both the inside and the outside. Topical applications (compresses, poultices, and steams) of astringent, anti-inflammatory, and antimicrobial herbs will clear and tone the skin directly. Internal preparations (tea, tincture, capsules) of liver-stimulating, circulatory-stimulant, and lymphatic herbs support the health and nourishment of skin tissue from beneath.

SKIN TONER

Makes 12 fluid ounces (90+ applications)

The acidity and probiotics from the vinegar combine with the astringency of the witch hazel and rose to gently but effectively tonify the skin, reducing blemishes and protecting against breakouts. Be consistent; results will begin to show after a few days to a week of use. This simple skin toner is a key part of Katja's vibrant skin protocol. (Though she's 44 years old, everyone thinks she's a decade younger.) If your skin is sensitive, reduce the amount of apple cider vinegar.

4 fluid ounces apple cider vinegar (preferably raw, unfiltered)
4 fluid ounces nonalcoholic witch hazel extract
4 fluid ounces rose water, or strong, well-strained rose petal infusion

1.In a small nonreactive bowl, stir together the vinegar, witch hazel, and rose water. This mixture is shelf stable. Store in an airtight container.
2.Apply this toner once a day after washing your face. If your skin tends toward dryness, rub a few drops of oil (rosehip or olive) into the skin afterward.
3.Apply this toner a second or third time during the day if your acne is persistent, but don't scrub too hard or use harsh soaps—just rinse gently with water first.

FACIAL STEAM

Makes 2 cups dried herb mix (4 to 8 steams)

For an active breakout, especially one that is oily, a steam is a great way to effectively deliver circulation-enhancing, inflammation-reducing, and bacteria-eliminating herbal action right into the pores.

½ cup dried chamomile flower
½ cup dried sage leaf
½ cup dried thyme leaf
½ cup dried yarrow leaf and flower
½ gallon water

1.In a small bowl, stir together the chamomile, sage, thyme, and yarrow. Store in an airtight container.
2.Clean your face with gentle soap and water.
3.Make and execute an herbal steam: In a medium pot over high heat, boil the water. Place the pot on a heat-proof surface, someplace where you can sit near it, and make a tent with a blanket or towel. Add ¼ to ½ cup of the herb mixture to the water. Position your face over the steam and remain there for 5 to 20 minutes. (Bring a tissue; the steam also clears your sinuses!)
4.Follow with spot applications of raw or herb-infused honey.

ACNE-FIGHTING TEA

1 cup Oregon grape root tea
50 drops yellow dock tincture

Combine the ingredients. Take up to one-third of the mixture three times daily.

ACNE WASH

1 cup horsetail tea
30 drops gotu kola tincture

Combine ingredients in a glass container with a lid. Use as much as needed to wash the skin, three times daily.

Aging

We all want to live to a ripe old age without looking a day over twenty-nine! Unfortunately, aging is a fact of life that occurs as the body's ability to function declines. The process of aging—marked by wrinkles, aching joints, fatigue, and loss or graying of hair—is accelerated by a poor diet, lack of exercise, excessive exposure to sunlight's ultraviolet rays, and lifestyle choices including smoking and drug use. These and other factors increase free-radical activity. Free radicals are highly unstable molecules that damage the cells' DNA and interfere with the cells' ability to function. A number of herbs function as antioxidants, which effectively eliminate free radicals.

Herbal Allies:
- Ginkgo biloba
- Ginger
- Parsley
- Milk thistle
- Black currants
- Elderberries
- Horsetail

ANTI-AGING TEA 1

½ cup Ginkgo biloba tea
½ cup ginseng tea

1. Combine the ingredients.
2. Take one-third of a cup three times daily.

Ginkgo is known to improve memory, while ginseng can boost energy levels.

ANTIAGING TEA 2

5 drops cayenne tincture
30 drops burdock tincture
15 drops goldenseal tincture
10 drops ginger root tincture
½ cup slippery elm tea (page 72)
1 cup warm water

1. Combine all ingredients.
2. Take 2 to 3 tablespoons three times per day to improve circulation.

Allergies

An allergy is a hypersensitive reaction to any of a number of substances. Allergies occur when the body's immune system malfunctions, going into "overdrive" to help protect the body from a substance it sees as foreign. Allergies are very common in the United States. In fact, more than one-third of all Americans suffer from an allergy of one type or another. Common symptoms include nasal congestion, coughing, watery eyes, sneezing, fatigue, and headaches. Some allergies may cause hives or an itchy rash. Severe allergies can cause the blood pressure to drop to dangerously low levels, leading to anaphylactic shock and death.

Hay fever is an acute type of allergy usually caused by airborne pollens. Trees and grasses are the typical culprits in this condition. Symptoms of hay fever include itchy eyes, mouth, and throat; watery eyes; sneezing; nasal discharge; and headaches.

Some people are allergic to molds, pollens, and dusts. Others react to certain foods such as wheat, milk, peanuts, eggs, or shellfish. Certain cosmetics or chemicals and even bee stings bring grief to many. The best way to treat an allergy is to avoid the offending substance. When that isn't possible, herbs can help check the watery eyes, nasal discharge, and coughing that occur with some allergics.

Relevant tissue states: heat (inflammation), laxity (of the mucous membranes)
Relevant herbal actions: antihistaminic, anti-inflammatory, kidney supportive, liver stimulant

Herbal Allies

- Agrimony
- All-heal leaf and flower
- Barberry Root
- Calendula flower
- Goldenrod leaf and flower
- Goldenseal
- Ground Ivy
- Marigold
- Milk thistle seed
- Mullein leaf
- Nettle leaf
- Oregon grape root
- Oxeye daisy
- Pearly everlasting flowers
- Plantain leaf
- Yerba sante

Allergic reactions to pollen, dust, or pets are primarily due to excessive histamine production, which ignites the inflammation underlying the runny nose, itchy eyes, and excessive phlegm. Histamine isn't all bad, though; it's a necessary part of sleep regulation, brain function, and even sexual response! Antihistaminic herbs are ideal because, while they help relieve allergy symptoms, they won't overshoot the mark and suppress histamine so much they cause adverse effects.

When trying to resolve allergies, we also must support the liver and kidneys. Among other things, the liver produces histaminase—an enzyme that breaks down histamine. So, when it's sluggish or overworked, histamine builds up and the inflammatory response worsens. The kidneys also help clear inflammatory instigators from the system, so giving them extra support helps reduce allergic symptoms.

ALLERGY RELIEF TEA

Makes about 3 to 4 cups dried herb mix (enough for 18 to 22 quarts of tea)

Nettle and goldenrod contain the antioxidant quercetin, which, according to a 2006 study by Shaik et al., stabilizes mast cells and prevents the release of histamine. Meanwhile, mullein supports the mucous membranes in the lungs and sinuses, reducing phlegm and mucus and quelling cough. Calendula and licorice improve liver function. Feel free to add some honey to your tea—especially if it's raw, local honey! Unfiltered honey helps reduce allergic response because it contains some pollen grains. Introducing these to the body through the oral route helps it become less reactive to them when you inhale pollen in the springtime.

1 cup dried nettle leaf (see Tips)
1 cup dried goldenrod leaf and flower
½ cup dried mullein leaf
½ cup dried calendula flower
½ to 1 cup marshmallow leaf (optional)
2 to 4 tablespoons dried licorice root

1.In a medium bowl, mix together all the herbs, including the marshmallow (if using, for a dry constitution). Store in an airtight container.
2.Make a long infusion: Prepare a kettle of boiling water. Measure 2 to 3 tablespoons of herbs per quart of water and place in a mason jar or French press. Pour in the boiling water, cover, and steep for 8 hours, or overnight.
3.Drink a quart or more every day, especially in the month before and during your personal peak allergy season. The earlier you start, the less you'll suffer.

TIP: Omit the nettle leaf and increase the goldenrod if you take blood-thinning pharmaceuticals.
TIP: Want a quick fix? No time for tea? The simple combination of freeze-dried nettle leaf capsules and milk thistle seed capsules offers quick relief from allergy. Choose a high-quality brand, and take 2 of each (with plenty of water) every 4 hours.

QUICK ALLERGY TEA

1 teaspoon barberry root
1 teaspoon Oregon grape root
1 cup water

1. Combine the herbs in a pan and cover with the water.
2. Bring to a boil. Reduce heat and simmer for 30 minutes. Strain.
3. Take one-third cup three times daily.

FLOWER DECOCTION

1 teaspoon oxeye daisy leaves
1 teaspoon pearly everlasting flowers
1 teaspoon yerba sante leaves
3 cups boiling water

1. Combine the herbs in a glass container and cover with the water; steep for 30 minutes; strain.
2. To use, take one-half to one cup every six hours.

NETTLE TEA

2 tablespoons nettle leaves
1 teaspoon Oregon grape root
2 cups boiling water

1. Combine all the herbs in a glass container and cover with the water; steep for 30 minutes; strain.
2. Take one-quarter cup three times a day.

Anemia

Anemia is a blood disorder marked by either red blood cells containing too little hemoglobin or too few red blood cells in the blood. (Hemoglobin is the protein in red blood cells that carries oxygen.) Anemia can have a number of causes, including alcoholism, excessive bleeding, illness, infections, poor bone marrow function, poor diet, and pregnancy. It is important to determine the cause of the anemia and treat the underlying condition.

Herbal Allies
- Barberry
- Oregon Grape Root
- Nettle

ANEMIA TEA

2 teaspoons barberry root
2 teaspoons Oregon grape root
4 tablespoons nettle leaves
2 cups cold water

1. Combine the herbs in a glass container.
2. Cover with the water.
3. Soak overnight.
4. Strain.
5. Take up to one-half cup three times daily.

Arthritis

There are two types of arthritis: rheumatoid arthritis and osteoarthritis. Rheumatoid arthritis (RA) is an autoimmune condition where the body sees itself as the enemy. The immune system's antibodies attack the joints and soft tissues, causing inflammation, pain, and gradual deterioration of the joint. RA can be a debilitating condition, especially when it occurs in young children.

Osteoarthritis is a degenerative disease, also called wear-and-tear arthritis. This form of arthritis affects many of us as we age. It occurs as the joints wear out over time. It usually starts in the joints of the hands and feet but eventually can affect even the larger joints of the body. Both rheumatoid arthritis and osteoarthritis can cause pain and stiffness.

In addition to the herbs listed below, other beneficial herbs for arthritis include bilberry, black currant, nettle, and vervain. The following treatments are effective for both osteoarthritis and rheumatoid arthritis.

Herbal Allies

- Balsam Bilberry
- Black Cohosh
- Black Currant
- Blue Vervain
- Cascara Sagrada
- Cayenne
- Chamomile
- Devil's Claw
- Feverfew
- Mullein
- Nettle
- Sarsaparilla
- White willow bark
- Wild Cherry
- Yucca

ARTHRITIS MILDING TEA

2 teaspoons devil's claw tuber
3 teaspoons white willow bark
1 teaspoon feverfew herb
2 teaspoons yucca root
2 teaspoons sarsaparilla root
3 cups cold water

1. Combine the herbs in a glass container and cover with the water.
2. Soak overnight.
3. Drain.
4. Take one-half cup three times daily.

QUICK ANALGESIC ARTHRITIS TEA

25 drops black cohosh tincture
90 drops wild cherry bark tincture
90 drops mullein tincture
1 cup warm water

1. Combine the above herbs in a glass container and cover with the water.
2. Take one-third of the mixture three times daily.

NIGHTLY ARTHRITIS TEA

1 teaspoon black cohosh root
1 teaspoon chamomile flowers
1 teaspoon cascara sagrada bark
2 cups water

1. Combine the above herbs in a glass container; cover with the water; stir thoroughly to combine.
2. Place 1½ teaspoons of the mixture in one cup boiling water; steep for 10 minutes; strain.
3. Take one cup in the evening, just before going to bed.

ARTHRITIS OINTMENT

1 pound petroleum jelly
1 tablespoon Canada balsam
2 tablespoons cayenne
2 tablespoons chamomile

1. Melt one pound of petroleum jelly in a double boiler.
2. Add herbs; stir; heat for 2 hours.
3. Remove from heat and strain by pouring the mixture through a cheesecloth, squeezing the cloth to release all the liquid.
4. While warm, pour the ointment into glass containers; cool.
5. Apply topically, massaging it until complete absorption, as needed for arthritis pain.

Asthma

If you've ever heard a child with asthma fighting for breath, you'll never forget the wheezing sound or the panic you feel as his or her skin begins to turn blue from lack of oxygen. Asthma is actually a common lung disease that affects people of all ages. In this disease, the trachea and bronchial tubes become inflamed. This causes the airways to narrow, restricting the flow of air, which in turn leads to shortness of breath, difficulty breathing, coughing, wheezing, and a tightness in the chest. An asthma attack can last from a few minutes to a few days and, if severe, can be life threatening.

No cause for the asthma can be determined for many people; however, for others, asthma attacks can be brought on by allergies to molds, pollen, or other allergens, as well as certain foods and drugs. Asthma can also be triggered by cold, damp weather; inhaling dust, smoke, or other irritants; and even infections. Unfortunately, asthma is on the upswing in this country, possibly because of the irritants in our polluted air.

Herbal allies

- Blue Vervain
- coltsfoot
- Echinacea
- Elecampane
- Ginseng
- Goldenseal

- Horehound
- Indian Root
- Passionflower
- Pleurisy root
- Wintergreen
- Yerba sante

QUICK-ACTING ASTHMA TEA

1 teaspoon elecampane root
2 teaspoons horehound herb
1 teaspoon blue vervain leaves
2 cups water

1. Combine the herbs in a pan and cover with water.
2. Bring to a boil; reduce heat and simmer for about 20 minutes; strain and cool.
3. Drink up to two cups a day, a mouthful at a time.

SOOTHING TEA

2 teaspoons powdered Indian root
2 teaspoons granulated echinacea root
2 teaspoons elecampane root
2 cups water

1. Combine the herbs in a pan and cover with the water.
2. Soak for several hours; strain.
3. Take one-half cup two times daily.

Back Pain

Back pain affects most of us at some time in our lives. It can be a dull ache or a sharp burning and stabbing. Sometimes back pain is accompanied by pain that radiates down your leg. This is called sciatica and is a sign that pressure is being placed on the nerves of the spinal cord. Sometimes back pain can be so severe that it limits your activities and renders you bedridden. Often, relaxing the muscles of the back can relieve back pain.

Back pain can have many causes—injury, spasms, sciatica (nerve pain), disc problems, and so on. Long-term resolution requires figuring out what exactly is the root of the problem, but in the meantime these herbs and formulas will relieve pain and release tension, allowing you to move more freely.

Relevant tissue states: tension (spasms), heat (inflammation)
Relevant herbal actions: analgesic, anti-inflammatory, antispasmodic, relaxant

Herbal Allies

- Barberry
- Black Cohosh
- Black Currant
- Black Haw
- Blue Cohosh
- Blue Vervain
- Devil's claw
- Echinacea
- Feverfew
- Ginger
- Goldenrod leaf and flower
- Meadowsweet flower
- Mullein root
- Solomon's seal root
- Wild lettuce

SPINE'S FINE TINCTURE

Makes 4 fluid ounces (40 to 120 doses)

These warming, relaxant, analgesic herbs quell the spasms responsible for most back pain, regardless of whether the pain is acute or chronic, muscular or connective, etc. If you have infused oil made from fresh goldenrod or ginger, use it as a massage oil after you apply this formula topically. For help sleeping, take 1 to 4 drops of tincture of wild lettuce by mouth—this will also contribute more pain-relieving action.

1 fluid ounce tincture of Solomon's seal
1 fluid ounce tincture of ginger
½ fluid ounce tincture of goldenrod
½ fluid ounce tincture of meadowsweet
½ fluid ounce tincture of mullein root (see Tip)
½ fluid ounce tincture of St. John's wort (optional; see Tip)

1.In a small bottle, combine the tinctures. Cap the bottle and label it.
2.Take 1 to 4 drops by mouth 3 to 5 times per day.
3.Additionally, squirt 1 to 4 drops into your palm and rub it into the back muscles.

TIP: If the vertebral discs are impinged or worn away, increase the mullein root to 1 fluid ounce. It specifically supports these tissues. If sciatica or other radiating nerve pain is present, include the tincture of St. John's wort (unless you are taking pharmaceuticals). It regenerates damaged nerve tissue.

WARMING COMPRESS

Makes 1 compress
This simple application provides immediate relief.

16 fluid ounces water
½ cup dried ginger (see Tip)
¼ cup Epsom salts

1.In a small pot with a tight-fitting lid over high heat, combine all the ingredients. Cover and bring to a boil. Reduce the heat and simmer for 5 minutes. Meanwhile, fill a hot water bottle.
2.Soak a cloth in the hot tea, holding it by a dry spot and letting it cool in the air until hot but comfortable to the touch.
3.Lie down and place the wet cloth over your back. Cover with a dry cloth and lay the hot water bottle on top. Get comfortable and let it soak in for 10 to 20 minutes. You should feel warmth, relaxation, and relief from pain.
4.Repeat as often as desired.

TIP: Have pain, but no dried ginger? If all you have on hand is fresh ginger from the grocery store, you can use that, too—sliced, chopped, or grated.

SCIATIC PAIN TEA

2 teaspoons crampbark
2 teaspoons kava kava root
2 cups water

1. Combine the herbs in a pan and cover with water.
2. Bring to a boil; reduce heat; simmer for 30 minutes.
3. Cool and strain.
4. Take up to one cup per day. This tea can help relieve sciatic pain.

ANALGESIC DAILY TEA FOR BACK PAIN

1 teaspoon coltsfoot leaves
2 teaspoons St. John's wort leaves
2 cups boiling water

1. Combine the herbs in a glass container and cover with boiling water; steep for 15 to 30 minutes; strain.
2. Take one-half cup in the morning and one-half cup at night.

SOOTHING BACK PAIN TEA

1 teaspoon chopped valerian root
2 teaspoons white willow bark
2 cups cold water

1. Combine the herbs in a pan and cover with the water.
2. Soak overnight; strain.
3. Take up to one cup a day, a tablespoon at a time.
This tea can help relieve pain caused by nerve irritation.

Bedsores

A bedsore, also called a decubitus ulcer, is an area of damage to the skin that can occur when pressure is applied to an area of the body for a prolonged period of time. The pressure restricts blood flow to the area and also causes irritation, leading to sores.

Skin ulcers are raw, open sores that occur when the top layer of skin cracks and peels away. They are marked by swelling, redness, pain, heat, and inflammation. They may also be infected and full of pus. Bedsores are very common in individuals in casts, as well as those confined to wheelchairs or to bed. In fact, the most common sites for bedsores are the lower back, the buttocks, and the heels. Some authorities estimate that treating bedsores and other decubitus ulcers costs the nation over $1 billion every year.

Herbal remedies

- Burdock
- Echinacea
- Evening primrose
- Marigold
- Nettle
- White Oak

BEDSORE TOPICAL WASH

2 teaspoons marigold flowers
1 teaspoon granulated echinacea root
1 tablespoon white oak bark
2 cups water

1. Combine the herbs in a glass container and cover with the water; soak overnight; strain.
2. Use as a wash periodically throughout the day.

Bites and Stings

Most of us have been bitten or stung by mosquitos, bees, wasps, ants, spiders, ticks, or even more exotic creatures, such as snakes or jellyfishes. We call it a "bite," but most insects and other creatures puncture the skin rather than actually take a bite. It is the substance the animal leaves in the wound and not the wound itself that usually does the damage.

Bites and stings frequently cause localized itching, pain, swelling, and redness. If untreated, any bite or sting can fester and become infected. Even though itching may be severe, resist the urge to scratch, as a secondary infection could result.

Native Americans have had thousands of years to practice using herbs on snakebites. Some of the most helpful herbs for this condition include echinacea and Seneca snakeroot.

Whether it's mosquitoes, black flies, or fire ants, most bug bites are fairly simple: We just need to reduce the inflammation. Bee and wasp stings are a bit more intense: Here, our goals include drawing out the venom, if possible, reducing inflammation, and helping the immune system cope with the venom that has entered the body. Watch for anaphylaxis! If someone stung or bitten is having difficulty breathing, seek help immediately.

Note: If you are stung by a bee or other pest and begin to feel weak, or if you notice any swelling anywhere on the body, call a physician immediately. You may be allergic to the sting and need emergency medical attention. Needless to say, if you are stung by a rattlesnake or other venomous snake, get immediate medical care.

Relevant tissue states: heat (inflammation)
Relevant herbal actions: anti-inflammatory, astringent, lymphatic, immune stimulant

Herbal Allies

- Echinacea
- Seneca snakeroot.
- Black currant
- Ginger
- Ginkgo biloba
- Licorice
- White willow
- Peppermint leaf
- Plantain leaf
- Rose
- Self-heal leaf and flower
- Yarrow leaf and flower

COOLING COMPRESS

Makes 1 compress

Peppermint's menthol provides a cooling sensation to the skin, while at the same time increasing blood circulation and dispersing the irritants from the bite or sting site.

16 fluid ounces water
½ cup dried peppermint leaf

¼ cup Epsom salts

1.In a small pot with a tight-fitting lid over high heat, combine all the ingredients. Cover and bring to a boil. Remove from the heat.
2.Soak a cloth in the hot tea, holding it by a dry spot and letting it cool in the air until hot but comfortable to the touch.
3.Apply the cloth to the bite or sting.

BUG BITE RELIEF SPRAY

Makes 8 fluid ounces (number of applications varies by use)

If you regularly walk through clouds of mosquitoes or black flies or live in an area infested with chiggers, you'll want this cooling, itch-relieving spray stocked for when you come inside.

4 fluid ounces nonalcoholic witch hazel extract or apple cider vinegar
2 fluid ounces tincture of rose
1 fluid ounce tincture of self-heal
1 fluid ounce tincture of yarrow

1.In a bottle with a fine-mist sprayer top, combine all the ingredients. Cap the bottle and label it.
2.Liberally spray wherever you've been bitten.

TOPICAL WASH FOR BITES AND STINGS

2 teaspoons comfrey leaves
2 tablespoons marshmallow leaves
1 tablespoon dried yarrow
1 cup boiling water

1. Combine the herbs in a nonmetallic container and cover with boiling water.
2. Steep for 15 to 30 minutes; strain.
3. Use as a topical wash.

SKIN SOOTHING OINTMENT

1 pound petroleum jelly
4 teaspoons dried agrimony leaves
4 teaspoons dried marigold flowers

1. Melt petroleum jelly in a double boiler.
2. Stir in the herbs and heat for 2 hours until the herbs begin to get crispy.
3. Strain by pouring through cheesecloth.
4. Squeeze the cloth to release all the liquid.
5. While warm, pour the ointment into clean glass containers. Use as needed.

Bronchitis

Bronchitis is an inflammation of the bronchial tubes that can range from a mild case (much like a bad cold) to a severe case, leading to pneumonia. Bronchitis may be accompanied by a fever, severe coughing, thick sputum, difficulty breathing, chills, and a sore throat. Bronchitis usually is caused by an infection but can also occur after inhaling dust, smoke, or other irritants. Repeated bouts of bronchitis can lead to chronic bronchitis, in which the bronchial tubes may become permanently damaged.

When you have a lung infection, don't suppress the cough—it's a vital response! Our goal is to cough when it's productive, so all the irritating or infectious material is expelled as you cough up phlegm, and to reduce the amount of unproductive coughing. If you can't bring up the phlegm, you may find a simple cough developing into pneumonia because of the mucus buildup. (True pneumonia is a serious condition—seek higher care. Meanwhile, take elecampane and garlic—they're your strongest allies for this problem.)

Infection-instigated coughs are usually wet, and the herbs we discuss here assume that's the case. The goal is to get it just a little on the moist side—nice and productive—so you can expel that phlegm.

As with any respiratory condition, an herbal steam is a great remedy all on its own, combating infection and greatly improving blood circulation—which means immune activity—in the lungs. A simple steam with thyme or sage is very good for this problem.

Relevant tissue states: dampness, cold (depressed vitality)
Relevant herbal actions: antimicrobial, astringent, decongestant, diaphoretic, expectorant, pulmonary tonic.

Herbal Allies

- Angelica
- Black Cohosh
- Black Elder
- Canadian fleabane
- Chamomile
- Coltsfoot
- Echinacea
- Elder
- Elecampane root
- Garlic
- Ginger
- Horehound
- Licorice
- Pearly Everlasting Flower
- Peppermint
- Pine
- Queen of the meadow
- Sage leaf
- Seneca snakeroot
- Slippery elm
- Thyme leaf

FIRE CIDER

Makes about 1 quart

Traditional fire cider recipes are blends of pungent and aromatic stimulating expectorants that will heat you up and help you get the gunk out. In this version, we sneak in some immune stimulants and a good source of vitamin C. Do not consume this if you take pharmaceutical blood thinners.

1 whole head garlic, cloves peeled and chopped
1 (2-inch) piece fresh ginger, chopped
¼ cup dried pine needles
¼ cup dried sage leaf
¼ cup dried thyme leaf
¼ cup dried elderberry
¼ cup dried rose hips
2 tablespoons dried elecampane root
2 tablespoons dried angelica root
1 quart apple cider vinegar
Honey or water, for sweetening or diluting (optional)

1. In a quart-size mason jar, combine the garlic, ginger, and remaining herbs.
2. Fill the jar with the vinegar. Cover the jar with a plastic lid, or place a sheet of wax paper under the jar lid before you screw down the ring. (The coating on the bottom of metal mason jar lids corrodes when exposed to vinegar.)
3. Let the herbs macerate in the vinegar for 2 weeks or longer.
4. Strain, bottle, and label the finished fire cider. If the vinegar is too heating to be comfortable on your stomach, add some honey (up to one-fourth the total volume), or dilute your dose with water.
5. Take a shot (about ½ fluid ounce) at the first sign of mucus buildup in the lungs, and every couple hours thereafter until symptoms resolve.

THROAT-SOOTHING TEA

2 teaspoons black cohosh root
2 teaspoons powdered Indian root
2 teaspoons chamomile flower
2 cups water
Honey, to taste

Combine the above herbs in a pan; cover with the water.
Bring to a boil; reduce heat and simmer for 30 minutes; strain.
Add honey if desired. Take one tablespoon in two cups of water several times a day.

SWEET SOOTHING TEA

1 teaspoon marshmallow leaves or flowers

1 teaspoon coltsfoot leaves
1 teaspoon mullein leaves and flowers
½ cup boiling water
Honey

Combine the above herbs; steep one teaspoon of the mixture in the boiling water; strain. Sweeten with honey. Take one-half cup, three or four times a day, hot.

BRONCHITIS TEA #3
1 teaspoon elecampane root
2 tablespoons nettle leaves
1 cup boiling water

Combine the above herbs. Pour the boiling water over the herbs and steep for 30 minutes; strain. Sweeten with honey, if desired. Take up to two cups a day.

BRONCHITIS TEA # 4
1 to 2 slices of fresh ginger root
1 teaspoon pearly everlasting flowers or leaves
1 teaspoon redroot
1 cup boiling water

Combine the above herbs; steep in the boiling water for 30 thirty minutes; strain. Take one-half cup of the tea, three times daily.

Burns and Sunburns

A burn is an injury to the skin or other tissues caused by fire (or another form of heat), electricity, chemicals, or radiation. Burns are classified according to their severity as first-degree, second-degree, or third-degree. In a first-degree burn, the skin will turn red and swell but will not blister. In a few days, there is complete healing, without scarring. The damage from a second-degree burn goes much deeper. The skin turns very red and there is blistering, although the skin heals without scarring. The most severe burn, third-degree, penetrates the skin, destroying both the epidermis and dermis (the segment of the skin beneath the epidermis). A third-degree burn can result in scar tissue formation. Burn tissue can become necrotic and also develop into a serious infection. Skin elasticity can be destroyed. A third-degree burn may actually be less painful than a more superficial first- or second-degree burn because nerve endings in the skin are destroyed. Burns can also occur internally from swallowing very hot liquids or inhaling hot air (such as that from a fire).

A severe burn can cause dangerous systemic damage, such as respiratory tract injury, infection, and shock. Anyone suffering from a severe burn should seek immediate medical attention to counter these potentially life-threatening effects. Herbs, however, can help relieve the pain from a minor burn and encourage rapid healing.

Relevant tissue states: heat
Relevant herbal actions: anti-inflammatory, antimicrobial, antiseptic, vulnerary

Herbal Allies

- Calendula flower
- Coneflower
- Echinacea
- Goldenrod
- Hyssop
- Linden leaf and flower
- Marshmallow
- Peppermint leaf
- Plantain leaf
- Rose petals
- Self-heal leaf and flower
- Sunflower
- Wild Indigo Root

Immediately following a burn, run cold water over the area—the skin retains heat for much longer than you'd expect. (If blisters form in the burned area, be very gentle with them and don't break them before they naturally slough off, if you can avoid it.) Then, gently clean the wound, removing any dirt or contaminant. Apply the herbs, combining antiseptics to prevent infection with cooling, wound-healing herbs to encourage tissue regeneration.

Apply any of the herbal allies in a wash, compress, poultice, or infused honey—don't use oily preparations (like salves) on burns, because they trap the heat in the tissue.

Do not underestimate the power of a marshmallow root poultice! Simply saturate a handful of marshmallow root with enough cold water to make a gloopy mass and apply it to the burn. Cover with gauze and leave in place for 20 minutes. Repeat frequently.

BURN-HEALING HONEY

Makes about 1 pint

Honey is the single best healing agent for burns: If you have nothing but plain honey, you're still in good shape. It gets even better, though, when you infuse these healing herbs into it ahead of time.

½ cup fresh calendula flower
½ cup fresh rose petals
1 pint honey, gently warmed

1.Put the calendula and rose petals in a pint-size mason jar.
2.Fill the jar with the warm honey. Seal the jar and place it in a warm area to infuse for 1 month.
3.In a double boiler, gently warm the closed jar until the honey has a liquid consistency. Strain the infused honey into a new jar, pressing the marc against the strainer to express as much honey as you can.
4.After cooling and cleaning a burn site, apply a layer of the infused honey and cover lightly with a gauze bandage. Refresh the application at least twice a day.

SUNBURN SPRAY

Makes 8 fluid ounces

A few spritzes cool the skin and begin to reduce inflammation.
1 tablespoon dried peppermint leaf
1 tablespoon dried plantain leaf
1 tablespoon dried self-heal leaf and flower
1 tablespoon dried linden leaf and flower
1 quart boiling water
4 fluid ounces rose water

1.Make a hot infusion: In a mason jar, combine the peppermint, plantain, self-heal, and linden. Pour in the boiling water, cover, and steep for 20 minutes.
2.Move the jar to the refrigerator until it's cold.
3.Strain out 4 fluid ounces of the infusion and transfer to an 8-ounce bottle with a fine-mist sprayer top. Use the remaining infusion for compresses or a cooling drink. It will keep, refrigerated, for 3 days.
4.Add the rose water to the spray bottle. Cap the bottle and label it.
5.Apply copiously and frequently. Keep the spray refrigerated when not in use.

BURN POULTICE

1 tablespoon dried coneflower flowers
1 tablespoon dried hyssop flowers

1 tablespoon dried goldenrod flowers
1 tablespoon dried sunflower petals

1. Combine the above ingredients; moisten with boiling water and place between two layers of cheesecloth; let cool and apply to the affected area.
2. When dry, remoisten. Use as often as necessary.

IMMUNITY STRENGTHENER

30 drops echinacea tincture
20 drops wild indigo root tincture
1 cup warm water

1. Combine the above herbs in the warm water.
2. Take up to five times a day.

A burn can weaken the body, leaving you vulnerable to illness and infection. Use this tea to strengthen immunity.

Canker Sores

Canker sores are small sores usually found on the lining of the mouth, although they can also occur on the lips, on the tongue, or in the throat. Also called aphthous ulcers, they can be white or yellow and are surrounded by red, inflamed tissue. These small ulcers can be extremely painful for several days and may be accompanied by fever and swollen lymph glands. Canker sores can be brought on by stress, viral infections, poor dental hygiene, and nutrient deficiencies. Injuries (such as certain dental procedures) can also cause canker sores to develop.

Herbal Allies
- Raspberries
- Black currants
- Big Sagebrush
- Echinacea
- Marigold

ANTI-INFLAMMATORY MOUTHWASH

½ cup barberry tea
½ cup white oak tea
½ cup echinacea tea
½ cup Oregon grape root tea

1. Combine the above ingredients in a glass container with a lid.
2. Use three times a day as a mouthwash. Be sure to swish the liquid around in your mouth for several minutes.

Cold Sores

Cold sores are small, painful, fluid-filled blisters on the mouth caused by the herpes simplex virus. Tingling, itching, and burning may give you a warning that a cold sore is about to erupt. The blisters may appear a few hours or days after the initial warning signs. After a few days, they eventually dry and form a crust. They usually completely heal within a week or two.

Relevant tissue states: heat (inflammation)
Relevant herbal actions: immune stimulant, lymphatic, vulnerary

Herbal Allies

- Burdock
- Echinacea
- Goldenseal
- White Oak
- Yerba Mansa
- Calendula flower

- Chamomile flower
- Linden leaf and flower
- Plantain leaf
- Self-heal leaf and flower
- St. John's wort leaf and flower
- Thyme leaf

COLD SORE COMPRESS

Makes 5 cups dried herb mix (about 50 applications)

This direct application stimulates local immunity and improves tissue quality so your body has the best chance to suppress the virus. For chicken pox or other full-body breakout, take an herb-infused bath with this same formula. Add a bit of baking soda, as it helps with the itching.

1 cup dried calendula flower
1 cup dried plantain leaf
1 cup dried chamomile flower
1 cup dried linden leaf and flower
½ cup dried self-heal leaf and flower
½ cup dried St. John's wort leaf and flower

1. In a large bowl, mix together all the herbs. Store in an airtight container.
2. Make a hot infusion: Prepare a kettle of boiling water. Measure 2 to 3 tablespoons of herbs per quart of water and place in a mason jar or French press. Pour in the boiling water, cover, and steep for 20 minutes. (Meanwhile, fill a hot water bottle.)
3. Soak a cloth in the warm tea, holding it by a dry spot and letting it cool in the air until hot but comfortable to the touch.
4. Lie down and place the wet cloth over the affected area. Cover with a dry cloth and lay the hot water bottle on top. Get comfortable and let it soak in for 10 to 20 minutes.
5. Repeat 2 to 3 times per day.

STEAM VARIATION: You can also perform a steam using these herbs as they're infusing. Simply make a blanket tent, position your face over the steaming pot, and steam yourself with these herbs for a few minutes before you sit with the compress.

COLD SORE BALM

Makes 5 ounces (about a 3-month supply)

This gentle salve is very soothing to irritated cold sores and helps reduce inflammation while making your body's environment less hospitable to the virus.

1 fluid ounce calendula-infused oil
1 fluid ounce plantain-infused oil
½ fluid ounce self-heal–infused oil
½ fluid ounce chamomile-infused oil
½ fluid ounce St. John's wort–infused oil
½ fluid ounce thyme-infused oil
1 ounce beeswax, plus more as needed

1. Make a salve as usual (see here for complete instructions). Make it nice and soft if you'll keep it in little jars; make it slightly firmer if you're using lip balm tubes.
2. Apply liberally to the affected area 3 to 5 times daily.

COLD SORE TEA

1 teaspoon burdock root
1 teaspoon dried and powdered goldenseal root
1 cup boiling water
Honey, to taste

1. Combine the above herbs in a glass container.
2. Pour the boiling water over the herbs; steep for 30 minutes, cool, and strain.
3. You may want to sweeten with honey. Take up to one cup a day.

COLD SORE MOUTHWASH

1 teaspoon echinacea root
1 teaspoon yerba mansa root
1 tablespoon white oak bark
1 cup boiling water

1. Combine the herbs in a glass container.
2. Pour the boiling water over the herbs.

3. Steep 30 minutes, cool, and strain. Use the solution as a wash to treat cold sores.

Constipation

Formerly called "costiveness," constipation refers to any irregularity in, or absence of, bowel movements. The frequency of bowel movements depends on your diet, your physical makeup, and your physical habits. Most people have one movement a day, but some people may go two days or more and not suffer from constipation. However, the longer waste products remain in the colon, the more water will be absorbed, and the drier and more compact the waste will become.

Constipation can occur because of a poor diet, inadequate water intake, nervous tension, insufficient exercise, drug use, poor or inconsistent toilet habits, and laxative overuse. A number of diseases, including thyroid problems, circulatory disorders, and colon disturbances (such as fistulas, inflammation, polyps, obstructions, and tumors) can also cause constipation.

Relevant tissue states: cold (stagnation), dryness, tension
Relevant herbal actions: bitter, carminative, demulcent, hepatic, laxative

Herbal Allies

- Angelica
- Barberry
- Boneset
- Cascara Sagrada
- Cayenne
- Chicory
- Dandelion root
- Ginger
- Marshmallow
- Milk thistle seed
- Oregon Grape
- St. John's wort leaf and flower
- Sunflower

Sometimes, constipation is simply a sign of dehydration—drink some water! If it's a chronic issue, it may be an indication of a food allergy or simply a sign that you're not getting sufficient fiber in your diet. A good, thick, cold infusion of marshmallow solves both problems: It rehydrates better than water alone, and it includes a lot of polysaccharides and fibers that help move stool along.

Constipation, especially when ongoing, can be traced back to sluggish liver function. Bile produced by the liver is a digestive fluid, but it also lubricates the intestines; when production is low, things can get stuck. Bitters and carminatives help spur digestive function, and liver-restorative herbs (hepatics) such as milk thistle can reestablish normal function.

BOWEL-HYDRATING INFUSION

Makes 2½ cups dried herb mix (enough for 14 to 18 quarts of tea)

A bit tastier than solo marshmallow, this is a great solution for the type of constipation that often afflicts people with dry constitutions. If you have hard-to-pass, dry, little "rabbit pellet" bowel movements, this is for you. Drink a quart or more every day.

1 cup dried linden leaf and flower

1 cup dried marshmallow root
¼ cup dried cinnamon bark
¼ cup dried licorice root

1.In a medium bowl, mix together all the herbs. Store in an airtight container.
2.Make a cold infusion: Measure 2 to 4 tablespoons of herbs per quart of water and place in a mason jar or French press. Pour in cold or room-temperature water and steep for 4 to 8 hours before straining.

BOWEL~MOTIVATING TINCTURE

Makes 4 fluid ounces (30 to 60 doses)

These bitters and carminatives will spur the bowels to movement by stimulating bile flow and intestinal peristalsis.

1½ fluid ounces tincture of dandelion root
1½ fluid ounces tincture of St. John's wort
½ fluid ounce tincture of angelica root
½ fluid ounce tincture of ginger

1.In a small bottle, combine the tinctures. Cap the bottle and label it.
2.Take 2 to 4 drops every 20 minutes until relief occurs.

BOWEL~SOOTHING TEA

One large handful of boneset flowers
One large handful of dandelion flowers
4 ounces cascara bark
2 quarts water
Honey

Combine the above herbs in a pan and cover with two quarts of water; bring to a boil; boil until the mixture reduces to one quart; strain.
Take one cup before breakfast and one at bedtime. You may want to add honey to sweeten.

PURIFYING DIGESTIVE TEA

2 teaspoons cascara sagrada
3 to 4 slices ginger root
1 teaspoon cayenne

1 teaspoon Oregon grape root
2 cups boiling water

Combine the above herbs in a pan and cover with two cups of boiling water; steep for 30 to 45 minutes, cool, and strain. Take one tablespoon at a time, up to two cups per day.

Cough and Cold

The common cold is an upper respiratory tract infection caused by one of more than 100 viruses. Symptoms of a common cold include watery eyes, runny or stuffy nose (rhinitis), head congestion (with a mild, moderate, or severe headache), fatigue, sneezing, and coughing. The cough that often accompanies a cold is the body's attempt to clear the air passage of mucus, dust, or other substances that cause irritation. Your sense of taste and smell may be decreased, and you may run a fever or suffer from chills. A general aching feeling of discomfort and listlessness (malaise) may be present. There may be a sore throat, ranging from mild to severe, as the cold develops. Any or all of these symptoms may be present.

Relevant tissue states: heat (irritation) or cold (depressed vitality), dryness or dampness
Relevant herbal actions: antitussive, astringent, decongestant, demulcent, diaphoretic, expectorant, pulmonary tonic

Herbal Allies

- Agrimony
- Black currant
- Black Elder
- Blue Vervain
- Boneset
- Chamomile
- Coltsfoot
- Echinacea
- Elecampane
- Fennel seed
- Ginger
- Gingko Biloba
- Goldenrod
- Goldenseal
- Horehound
- Indian Root
- Licorice
- Mullein
- Osha
- Oxeye Daisy
- Peppermint
- Pine
- Pleurisy Root
- Queen of the Meadow
- Speedwell
- White cedar leaf tips
- Wild Cherry
- Wild Indigo
- Yarrow
- Yerba mansa
- Yerba sante
- Marshmallow
- Mullein leaf
- Sage leaf
- Thyme leaf

For herbs to work best, we need to differentiate between a hot, dry, irritated cough and one that is wet, but cold and unproductive. When the lungs are dry, you'll have a racking, relentless cough; we use moistening herbs to correct this. Wet lungs rattle or gurgle and are most likely a response to infection. See Bronchitis/Chest Cold/Pneumonia or Cold and Flu.

LUNG~LUBRICATING TEA

Makes 2¾ cups dried herb mix (enough for 18 to 22 quarts of tea)

For dry, hot lungs, these soothing and moistening herbs bring relief from a racking, unrelenting cough.

1 cup dried marshmallow root
1 cup dried mullein leaf
½ cup fennel seed
¼ cup dried licorice root, or to taste
Honey, for extra soothing (optional)

1. In a medium bowl, mix together all the herbs. Store in an airtight container.
2. Make a cold infusion: Measure 2 to 4 tablespoons of herbs per quart of water and place in a mason jar or French press. Pour in cold or room-temperature water and steep for 4 to 8 hours.
3. Strain the liquid and drink directly, or warm, if desired.
4. Add honey (if using) for extra soothing.

ANTITUSSIVE OXYMEL

Makes about 1 quart (20 to 60 doses)

An oxymel is simply a blend of vinegar and honey, which combines the astringent and stimulating effects of the vinegar with the moistening and soothing aspects of the honey. Adding lung-specific herbs makes this a go-to for coughs of all kinds.

⅓ cup dried pine needles
⅓ cup dried sage leaf
⅓ cup dried thyme leaf
¼ cup dried ginger
1 quart apple cider vinegar
Honey, as needed for topping off the jar

1. In a quart-size mason jar, combine the herbs.
2. Fill the jar four-fifths full with vinegar; top off with honey.
3. Cover the jar and let macerate for 4 weeks.
4. Strain and bottle the oxymel. Cap the bottle and label it.
5. Take 1 to 3 tablespoons as needed.

COUGH SYRUP

2 teaspoons coltsfoot leaves
1 tablespoon wild plum root
2 teaspoons mullein leaves
2 cups boiling water
1 pound honey

1. Combine the above herbs in the boiling water; in a nonmetallic container steep for 30 minutes and strain.
2. Add one pound of honey, heating and stirring until the honey is dissolved; cool and store in a glass container.
3. Take one tablespoon at a time, as needed.

SOOTHING COUGH AND COLD FORMULA

30 drops echinacea tincture
20 drops wild indigo root tincture
2 cups white cedar leaf tips tea

1. Combine the above ingredients and take half a cup at a time, hot.
2. Take up to three times a day.

LAKOTA COUGH AND COLD FORMULA

1 teaspoon goldenseal root
1 teaspoon mullein leaves
1 teaspoon osha root
1 teaspoon pleurisy root
1 teaspoon yerba mansa root
2 teaspoons yerba sante leaves
2 cups boiling water

1. Combine the above herbs and cover with the boiling water; steep for 30 minutes, cool, and strain.
2. Take two tablespoons at a time, as needed, up to two cups a day.

LUMBEE COUGH AND COLD FORMULA

3 teaspoons goldenrod leaves

4 teaspoons horehound leaves
2 teaspoons white pine inner bark
4 cups boiling water

1. Combine the above herbs in a cheesecloth; tie closed with a string.
2. Place the bag in the boiling water; boil for 15 minutes; cool; remove the bundle.
3. Take half a cup of the hot mixture at a time, as needed, up to two cups a day.

QUICK~ACTING COUGH AND COLD FORMULA

4 teaspoons agrimony leaves
2 teaspoons mullein leaves
2 teaspoons blue vervain leaves
1 teaspoon oxeye daisy
3 teaspoons horehound leaves
2 teaspoons speedwell
2 cups boiling water

1. Combine the above herbs in a nonmetallic container and cover with the boiling water; steep for 30 minutes, cool, and strain.
2. Take a tablespoonful every three hours, as needed, up to two cups a day.

EXPECTORATING COUGH AND COLD TEA

2 teaspoons boneset herb
2 teaspoons licorice root
2 to 3 slices ginger root
2 teaspoons wild cherry bark
2 cups boiling water

Combine the above herbs in a nonmetallic container and cover with the boiling water; steep for 30 minutes, cool, and strain. Take one to two tablespoons at a time, up to two cups a day, as needed, for a dry tickling cough.

DECONGESTANT TEA

2 slices fresh ginger
2 teaspoons pleurisy root
1 cup boiling water

1. Combine the herbs in a glass container; pour one cup of boiling water over the herbs; steep for 30 minutes, cool, and strain.
2. Take a tablespoon at a time, up to two cups a day. This tea is good for bronchial congestion.

ANTITUSSIVE FLOWER TEA

1 teaspoon elderflowers
1 teaspoon yarrow flowers
1 cup boiling water

1. Combine the herbs in a nonmetallic container and cover with one cup of boiling water; steep for 20 minutes and strain.
2. Drink hot every two hours, as needed.

QUICK~ACTING MULLEIN COUGH SYRUP

1 cup of mullein tea
1 pound honey

1. Combine the above ingredients in a pan and heat until the honey is liquid.
2. Remove from heat, cool, and pour into a glass container. Take a tablespoon at a time, as needed.

ELECAMPANE COUGH SYRUP

2 cups of elecampane tea
1 pound honey

1. Combine the tea with the honey and heat on low. Stir to dissolve the honey; when dissolved, remove the mixture from the heat.
2. When cool, pour into glass containers and seal.
3. Take two tablespoons at a time, as needed, up to one cup a day.

HOREHOUND LOZENGES

1½ cups horehound leaves
1½ cups water

3 cups sugar
3 tablespoons corn syrup

1. Place the horehound leaves in a pan and cover with the water.
2. Bring the mixture to a boil and boil for 20 minutes.
3. Remove from the heat and cool. Strain the solution and add the sugar and corn syrup.
4. Place back on the heat, bring to a boil, then reduce heat to medium.
5. Cook until the mixture reaches 300°F (hard-crack stage).
6. Pour the syrup onto a large buttered baking sheet; cool, then break into one-inch pieces.
7. Use as you would any cough drop.

Cramps

Cramping muscles are involuntary muscle contractions. They can be very painful and tight. Muscle cramps can be caused by cold temperatures, dehydration, overexercise, nutrient imbalances, and restricted blood flow to the muscles. Muscle cramps also can be caused by an imbalance in the body's electrolytes (electrolytes in the body include calcium, magnesium, potassium, and sodium). Muscle cramps usually occur in the legs, where they can often be severe enough to keep you from walking. Muscle cramps can also occur in the arms, the back, and in virtually any and every muscle of the body.

Relevant tissue states: heat (inflammation), tension
Relevant herbal actions: anodyne, nervous tropho-restorative, relaxant, rubefacient

Herbal Allies

- Black Cohosh
- Ginseng
- Wintergreen
- Yerba Mansa
- Cinnamon bark
- Ginger
- Goldenrod leaf and flower
- Meadowsweet flower
- Peppermint essential oil
- Wild lettuce
- Yarrow leaf and flower

A bit of delayed-onset muscle soreness after a hard day's work or an intense workout is normal. Rest well! Recovery time is when muscles grow stronger; if you don't give them time to recover fully, you'll confound your efforts. Eat well, too: providing the necessary nutrients speeds recovery. Bone broth with seaweed added is a great place to start.

MUSCLE~WARMING OINTMENT

20 drops yerba mansa tincture
4 ounces wintergreen oil
1 pound petroleum jelly

1. Thoroughly mix the above herbs with the petroleum jelly.
2. Use as an ointment to relieve muscle cramps.

MUSCLE CRAMP TEA

2 teaspoons black cohosh root
1 tablespoon ginseng root
2 cups water

1. Combine the above herbs in a pan and cover with two cups of water; bring to a boil; reduce heat and simmer for 30 minutes, cool, and strain.
2. Take two to three tablespoons up to six times a day.

MUSCLE RUB

Makes 8 fluid ounces (100+ applications, 30-day supply)

These warming herbs increase local circulation, simultaneously reducing inflammation and soothing tension. If, after applications, you're still in a lot of pain when it's time to go to bed, take 1 to 2 drops of wild lettuce tincture for further relief.

2 fluid ounces ginger-infused oil
2 fluid ounces goldenrod-infused oil
2 fluid ounces tincture of ginger
2 fluid ounces tincture of meadowsweet
80 drops peppermint essential oil or cinnamon essential oil (or both!)

1. In a small bottle, combine the infused oils, tinctures, and essential oil(s). Cap the bottle and label it, including Shake well before each use.
2. Hold your palm over the bottle's mouth and tilt to deposit a small amount in your palm. Rub between your hands to warm the treatment, and apply to the painful joints.
3. Massage the liniment into the joints until your hands no longer feel oily. Really work the liniment into the tissue.
4. Repeat the application 3 to 5 times per day. More is better!

DIARRHEA

Diarrhea is marked by frequent and excessive discharge of watery fecal material. Diarrhea can occur because of bacterial or viral infections or intestinal parasites. Certain chemicals and drugs can cause diarrhea, as can certain diseases, such as ulcerative colitis and cancer. Emotional stress can also bring on diarrhea. Food allergies, drinking caffeine or alcohol, or eating unripe fruit or spoiled food can also bring on an attack.
Excessive or prolonged diarrhea can cause dehydration, which can interfere with the absorption of nutrients. Diarrhea can be especially dangerous in children because they cannot tolerate much fluid loss.

Relevant tissue states: laxity (barrier compromise), dampness
Relevant herbal actions: astringent, demulcent

Herbal Allies

- Agrimony
- Alumroot
- Angelica
- Barberry
- Blackberry
- Black Currant

- Canadian fleabane
- Catnip
- Cayenne
- Cinnamon bark
- Ginger Root
- Marshmallow
- Meadowsweet flower
- Mint
- Pine Bark
- Plantain leaf
- Raspberry
- Rose
- Self-heal leaf and flower
- Strawberry leaf
- Witch hazel
- Yarrow
- Yellow Dock

When the lining of the bowels loses integrity, excess fluid is lost. To counteract this directly, astringent herbs restore healthy tone to the mucous membranes, so water stays in the body where it belongs. Once this is accomplished, it's a good idea to follow up with some soothing demulcent herbs—especially if the diarrhea has been going on for a while, as that causes dehydration, which must be corrected.

ASTRINGENT TEA

Makes 2¼ cups dried herb mix (enough for 14 to 18 quarts of tea)

The tannins in these herbs help bind lax tissues back together so fluids stay where they belong and barriers keep their integrity. Drink a quart of tea over the course of the day.

1½ cups dried self-heal leaf and flower
½ cup dried meadowsweet flower
¼ cup rose petals

1. In a medium bowl, mix together all the herbs. Store in an airtight container.
2. Make a hot infusion: Prepare a kettle of boiling water.
3. Measure 2 to 3 tablespoons of herbs per quart of water and place in a mason jar or French press.
4. Pour in the boiling water, cover, and steep for 20 minutes or until cool enough to drink.

TINCTURE VARIATION: If you prefer, make a tincture blend using the same proportions: Combine 1½ fluid ounces tincture of self-heal, ½ fluid ounce tincture of meadowsweet, and ¼ fluid ounce tincture of rose petal. Take 1 to 6 drops every 20 minutes until relief occurs.

CINNAMON POWDER CAPSULES

Makes 20 to 24 capsules

When cinnamon is extracted into water—as an infusion or decoction—its demulcent quality is emphasized. However, if you swallow a capsule of the powder, the capsule dissolves in your GI tract and releases the dry powder, which then absorbs excess water and exerts an astringent effect on the intestinal lining. This quells diarrhea quite nicely. The Capsule Machine, a handy manual capsule-filling device, helps with this recipe quite a lot.

20 to 24 empty gelatin capsules, size "00"
2 tablespoons powdered cinnamon

1. Fill the capsules with the cinnamon powder.
2. Take 1 to 3 capsules when you have diarrhea. If relief isn't obtained within an hour, take another dose.

QUICK AND EASY DIARRHEA TEA

3 tablespoons agrimony leaves
2 tablespoons self-heal
4 cups water

1. Combine the herbs in a pan; cover with the water; bring to a boil; reduce heat and simmer for 30 minutes; cool and strain.
2. Drink as needed, up to one cup a day.

SOOTHING DIARRHEA TEA

2 teaspoons alumroot
2 teaspoons blackberry leaves
2 teaspoons angelica seeds
1 teaspoon Oregon grape root
2 cups boiling water

1. Combine the above herbs in a nonmetallic container.
2. Pour the boiling water over the herbs and steep for 30 minutes; strain; take as needed, up to one cup a day.

IROQUOIS TEA

2 teaspoons raspberry leaves
2 teaspoons strawberry leaves

2 tablespoons yarrow
2 teaspoons yellow dock root
2 cups boiling water

1. Combine the herbs in a glass container; pour the boiling water over the herbs; steep for 30 minutes; cool and strain.
2. Take up to one cup a day. The Iroquois made a similar tea to treat bloody diarrhea.

Fatigue

Fatigue is more than just being tired. Instead, fatigue is a prolonged or excessive decrease in the ability to function, over and above what normal exertion would cause. Those who push themselves to the point of physical exhaustion are certainly familiar with fatigue. However, fatigue can be a symptom of more than overexertion; it is a symptom of a number of conditions including anemia, circulatory problems (such as angina pectoris, atherosclerosis, and high blood pressure), chronic fatigue syndrome, diabetes, hepatitis, inflammatory bowel disease, multiple sclerosis, and respiratory conditions including pneumonia and pleurisy.

Relevant tissue states: cold (depletion, depression, exhaustion)
Relevant herbal actions: adaptogen, exhilarant, stimulant

Herbal Allies

- Angelica
- Ashwagandha root
- Blackberry
- Gingko Biloba
- Ginseng
- Gotu Kola
- Licorice root
- Mirabilis
- Pulsatilla
- Raspberry
- St. John's Wort
- Strawberry leaf
- Tulsi leaf

Fatigue is an indication that something is impairing recovery. Most of the time, it's simply a lack of sleep. (Believe it or not, healthy adults need 8 to 10 hours of sleep a night—every night—and most Americans only get 6 on weekdays, 8 on weekends!) Even if your fatigue is not immediately relieved by a good night's sleep, it's still important to prioritize sleep. While there can be other factors in play (malnutrition, chronic illness, stress, pharmaceutical side effects, etc.), sleep is irreplaceable.

To counter fatigue, we should not underestimate the importance of movement for building energy. A little bit of motion can grow into greater kinetic energy if you cultivate it, gently and consistently. Tai chi and qigong are excellent for this.

While you're working on that, we'll draw on the talents of our adaptogens and uplifting, stimulating herbs to help break through the fog and push forward.

SHAKE-IT-OFF FORMULA

Makes 3 fluid ounces (45 to 90 doses)

1 fluid ounce tincture of licorice
1 fluid ounce tincture of ashwagandha
1 fluid ounce tincture of tulsi

1. In a small bottle, combine the tinctures. Cap the bottle and label it.

2.Take 1 to 2 drops, at morning and noontime. Feel free to take additional doses whenever you need a boost.

UP~AND~ABOUT MORSELS

Makes about 24 pieces

These tasty, restorative treats are a good way to get a substantial dose of beneficial herbs. This format is particularly useful because it provides the full complement of plant compounds instead of just those that are water soluble or alcohol soluble, as happens with a tea or tincture.

¼ cup powdered ashwagandha root
¼ cup powdered tulsi leaf
¼ cup powdered milk thistle seed
¼ cup powdered nettle leaf
3 tablespoons powdered licorice root
¾ cup nut butter
½ cup honey

Unsweetened shredded coconut, cocoa powder, powdered cinnamon, powdered ginger, cayenne, or whatever seems tasty to you, for coating

1.In a large bowl, blend the powders together.
2.Add the nut butter and honey. Stir to form a thick "dough."
3.Roll the dough into balls about the size of a walnut (1 inch).
4.Roll the balls in your coating of choice.
5.Eat 1 to 4 per day.

PICK~ME~UP TEA

1 teaspoon Ginkgo biloba leaves
1 teaspoon dried mirabilis root
1 teaspoon dried ginseng root
1 teaspoon pulsatilla herb
1 teaspoon gotu kola leaves
1 teaspoon St. John's wort leaves
4 cups boiling water

1. Combine the above herbs in a glass container; cover with the boiling water; steep for 30 minutes; strain.
2. Take as needed.

INVIGORATING TEA

1 teaspoon blackberry leaves
1 teaspoon strawberry leaves
1 teaspoon raspberry leaves
2 cups boiling water
Honey

1. Combine the above herbs in a glass container; cover with the boiling water; steep for 10 minutes; strain.
2. Sweeten with honey if desired. Drink as needed.

Fever

"Normal" body temperature is generally considered to be 98.6°F, although that number may vary between individuals, or even in the same individual at different times of the day. For example, our body temperature is lowest in the early morning and highest in the late afternoon. However, a fever is considered to be any temperature above 100°F. A fever is usually a sign that the body is fighting off some type of infection.

Whether or not to treat a fever is a very controversial subject. In my opinion, fever is the body's way of repairing itself and should not be suppressed. However, fever in children and in adults with heart illness and other disorders is sometimes serious and may need to be treated.

Relevant tissue states: heat, dryness (dehydration)
Relevant herbal actions: diaphoretic, refrigerant

Herbal Allies

- Angelica
- Boneset
- Cayenne
- Catnip leaf and flower
- Elderflower
- Garlic
- Ginger
- Juniper
- Marigold
- Osha Root
- Oxeye Daisy
- Peppermint leaf
- Sage leaf
- Skullcap
- Thyme leaf
- Tulsi leaf
- Wild Indigo Root
- Wild lettuce
- Yarrow leaf and flower

Fever is your friend: It's a vitally important immune response—and herbalists aren't the only ones saying so! The American Academy of Pediatrics released a clinical report in 2011 that stated: "It should be emphasized that fever is not an illness but is, in fact, a physiologic mechanism that has beneficial effects in fighting infection." So, don't give in to fever phobia—help your body do its work.

Stay hydrated! Almost all serious problems associated with fever come not from the fever itself but from runaway dehydration. If a person is too nauseous to keep down fluids, sitting in a warm bath is a good way to rehydrate.

Finally, remember that temperatures are relative to individuals. Children run hot, elders run cool, and constitution influences your baseline body temperature. A limp and unresponsive person at 99°F is in more trouble than an active, alert person at 101°F. So, always look at the person more closely than the thermometer.

FEVER~INDUCING TEA

Makes 3 cups dried herb mix (enough for 18 to 24 quarts of tea)

Often we want to help fever come on strong, with the help of our stimulating diaphoretics. These will help a fever be more productive, and they can also help the fever be more bearable because they cause the body to sweat. Drink a big mug of this tea whenever a fever is low and lingering and you want to boost it into an effective heat.

1 cup dried tulsi leaf
½ cup dried sage leaf
½ cup dried thyme leaf
½ cup dried yarrow leaf and flower
¼ cup dried angelica root
¼ cup dried ginger
1 garlic clove, sliced, for a real kick (optional)

1. In a medium bowl, mix together all the herbs. Store in an airtight container.
2. Make a hot infusion: Prepare a kettle of boiling water. Measure 2 to 3 tablespoons of herbs per quart of water and place in a mason jar or French press. Add the garlic (if using). Pour in the boiling water, cover, and steep for 20 minutes.
For best effect, reheat before drinking and drink very hot.

FEVER~BREAKING TEA

Makes 1¾ cups dried herb mix (enough for 14 to 24 pints of tea)

If the fever is too hot to tolerate, these relaxing diaphoretics and refrigerants will relieve tension and release the heat without stimulating more fire. The wild lettuce in the mix will make you sleepy, which is good—sleep is your best healing mechanism. Go to bed!

½ cup dried catnip leaf and flower
½ cup dried elderflower
½ cup dried peppermint leaf
¼ cup dried wild lettuce leaf and stalk
1 pint boiling water

1.In a medium bowl, mix together all the herbs. Store in an airtight container.
2.Make a hot infusion: Measure 1 to 2 tablespoons of herbs and place in a pint-size mason jar. Pour in the boiling water, cover, and steep for 20 minutes or until cool. Drink this tea slightly cooler than usual.
3.Sip on a mugful when you want to reduce a fever.

FEVER RELIEF TEA

1 teaspoon angelica root
1 teaspoon ground ivy leaves
1 teaspoon barberry berries
2 teaspoons peppermint leaves
2 teaspoons blue vervain leaves
1 tablespoon dried yarrow
1 teaspoon catnip leaves
1 cup boiling water

1. Combine the above herbs.
2. Place one tablespoon of the mixture in a cup; pour the boiling water over the herbs; steep for 30 minutes; strain.
3. Take up to one cup a day.

QUICK-ACTING FEVER TEA

1 teaspoon echinacea root
1 teaspoon white willow root
1 cup water

1. Combine the roots in a pan and cover with the water.
2. Bring to a boil; reduce heat and simmer for 30 minutes; cool and strain.
3. Take half a cup, up to four times a day.

Food Intolerances

Food sensitivities are extremely common and run the gamut from mild to life-threateningly severe. They cause all manner of gastrointestinal upsets—heartburn, IBS, bloating, and more—but can also contribute to systemic inflammation, neurological problems, and autoimmunity. In our opinion, everyone should periodically assess for sensitivity to a few common foods: Gluten, dairy, soy, corn, eggs, and nightshades (potatoes, tomatoes, peppers, eggplant, etc.) are all common culprits. A 30-day elimination period similar to what's described on Whole30.com, during which you avoid the suspect food entirely and track the severity of your symptoms, is the best way to identify if you have a sensitivity to a particular food.

Once your individual trigger foods are identified and eliminated from your diet, there's still some cleanup and reset work to do—that's where herbs really shine. A cup or two of herb-infused broth and a quart of gut-healing infusion in a day will have you feeling like a new person in no time.

Relevant tissue states: heat (inflammation), laxity (barrier compromise)
Relevant herbal actions: bitter, carminative, demulcent, hepatic, nervine, nutritive, relaxant, vulnerary

Herbal Allies

- Angelica
- Barberry
- Bayberry
- Blue Cohosh
- Calendula flower
- Catnip leaf and flower
- Chamomile flower
- Coneflower
- Dandelion
- Echinacea
- Fennel seed
- Ginger
- Kelp
- Licorice root
- Marshmallow
- Meadowsweet flower
- Oregon grape
- Peppermint
- Plantain leaf
- Self-heal leaf and flower
- St. John's wort leaf and flower
- Tulsi leaf
- Yarrow leaf and flower

Flatulence, or gas, is often a symptom of indigestion and can develop when we eat too fast or too much. It can also occur because of allergies or enzyme deficiencies and is a sign that our bodies are not breaking down the foods that we eat. For example, those people whose bodies do not make the enzyme lactase can't adequately digest the sugars in dairy products. The milk sugars in these products then ferment in the colon, causing gas. High-fiber foods can also cause flatulence, as can beans and cabbage.

Indigestion refers to any gastrointestinal disturbance, such as an upset stomach. Indigestion can occur if you eat too fast, eat too much, eat while emotionally upset, or, for some people, eat the wrong foods. Caffeine, high-fiber foods, alcohol, and carbonated drinks are often indigestion culprits. Sometimes allergies can cause indigestion. Indigestion can be a symptom of a number of diseases, including pancreatitis, ulcers, gastritis, and cholecystis. Often, however, there is no known cause for indigestion.

GUT~HEAL TEA

Makes 4⅓ cups dried herb mix (enough for 20 to 40 quarts of tea)

This blend of digestive herbs combines all the actions needed to restore healthy function to the stomach, intestines, and liver. It is the single most-frequently recommended formula in our practice and is open to a wide degree of individual customization: If you have lots of gut cramping, add more chamomile and fennel. If you're constitutionally dry, add more marshmallow. If you run very hot, omit the ginger. If there's an herb you don't like, just leave it out, and if there's one you particularly love, add more! Drink a quart or more every day.

½ cup dried calendula flower
½ cup dried plantain leaf
½ cup dried chamomile flower
½ cup dried tulsi leaf
⅓ cup dried catnip leaf and flower
⅓ cup fennel seed
⅓ cup dried peppermint leaf
⅓ cup dried marshmallow leaf
¼ cup dried ginger
¼ cup dried licorice root
¼ cup dried yarrow leaf and flower
¼ cup dried St. John's wort leaf and flower (see Tip)

1. In a large bowl, mix together all the herbs. Store in an airtight container.
2. Make a hot infusion: Prepare a kettle of boiling water. Measure 2 to 3 tablespoons of herbs per quart of water and place in a mason jar or French press. Pour in the boiling water, cover, and steep for 20 minutes or until cool enough to drink.
TIP: Omit the St. John's wort if you are concurrently taking pharmaceuticals.

BUILD~UP BROTH

Makes about 3 quarts

Bone broth is very healing to the gut, especially when the bones have bits of collagen (gristle) attached. The amino acids in these parts help restore intestinal integrity, which is compromised by the food allergy reaction. Adding herbs enhances these healing and anti-inflammatory activities. If you feel particularly awful, forego solid food for a day and just have lots of broth! One more reason to get in the bone broth habit: Broth made from bones with collagenous tissue still attached is rich in glucosamine and chondroitin. These nutrients are utilized by the body to rebuild healthy joints and connective tissues. You can buy glucosamine and chondroitin as supplements, but bone broth is a cheaper source and has so many other additional benefits!

1 cup dried calendula flower

¼ cup dried dandelion root
¼ cup fennel seed
¼ cup dried ginger
¼ cup dried kelp
Bones (such as from 1 rotisserie chicken; 6 pork chop bones; 1 lamb or beef shank; or the bones, head, and tail from 2 medium fish—really, any bones will do . . .)
3 quarts water, plus more as needed
1 tablespoon apple cider vinegar
Oyster, shiitake, or maitake mushrooms, for their nutritive and healing properties (optional)
Salt
Freshly ground black pepper

1. In a large pot over high heat, combine the herbs, bones, water, vinegar, and mushrooms (if using). Season with salt and pepper. Bring to a boil. Sustain boiling for 4 to 8 hours. Check often and add enough water to replace what has boiled away.
2. Strain the liquid and reserve. Compost the bones and herb marc, if desired.
3. Drink a mug of warm broth 2 to 3 times per day.

STOP~FLATULENCE TEA

1 teaspoon dried angelica root
2 teaspoons peppermint leaves
1 teaspoon bee balm leaves
1 cup boiling water

1. Combine the herbs in a container.
2. Take one tablespoon of the herb mixture and cover with the boiling water; steep for 20 to 30 minutes; strain. Take as needed.

COLON~SOOTHING TEA

2 teaspoons bee balm leaves
2 teaspoons peppermint leaves
2 teaspoons chamomile flowers
1 cup boiling water

1. Combine the herbs in a container.
2. Take one tablespoon of the mixture and cover with the boiling water; steep for 30 minutes; strain. Take as needed.

QUICK-ACTING FLATULENCE TEA

1 teaspoon catnip leaves
1 teaspoon grated ginger root
2 teaspoons dandelion leaves
2 cups boiling water

1. Combine the herbs and cover with the boiling water; steep for 20 to 30 minutes; strain.
2. Take as needed.

GUT-CLEARING TEA

1 teaspoon blue cohosh root
1 teaspoon coneflower root
1 cup boiling water

1. Combine the above herbs in a glass container.
2. Pour the boiling water over the herbs; steep for 30 minutes; cool and strain. Take as needed, up to one cup a day.

DAILY DIGESTIVE TEA

1 teaspoon angelica root
1 teaspoon grated ginger root
2 teaspoons chamomile flowers
2 teaspoons peppermint leaves
1 cup boiling water

1. Combine the above ingredients in a container.
2. Take one tablespoon of the herb mixture and place in the boiling water; steep for 30 minutes; cool and strain. Take as needed, up to two cups a day.

PEPPERY INDIGESTION TEA

1 teaspoon licorice root
1 teaspoon peppermint leaves
2 cups boiling water

1. Combine the above herbs in a nonmetallic container and cover with the boiling water; steep for 15 to 20 minutes; strain.
2. Take as needed, up to one cup a day.

Hangover

Everyone knows what a hangover is, even if they have never experienced one firsthand. Excessive alcohol intake dehydrates the body, which is why those suffering from a hangover have a dry mouth and are thirsty. Too much alcohol can also elevate and then drastically drop blood sugar levels, leading to headache, irritability, shakiness or dizziness, and fatigue. Alcohol depletes the body of certain nutrients and can cause fat to build up in the liver. It also causes the stomach to excrete too much acid, which can lead to heartburn, nausea, and vomiting. No wonder a hangover feels so awful.

Relevant tissue states: heat (inflammation), dryness (dehydration), laxity (barrier compromise)
Relevant herbal actions: anodyne, antiemetic, anti-inflammatory, relaxant

Herbal Allies

- Barberry
- Bayberry
- Betony leaf and flower
- Catnip
- Chaparral
- Chamomile flower
- Ginger
- Goldenseal
- Linden leaf and flower
- Licorice root
- Marshmallow
- Milk thistle seed
- Oregon Grape
- Plantain leaf
- Peppermint
- Self-heal leaf and flower
- St. John's wort leaf and flower

The number-one hangover preventive and simplest remedy is milk thistle capsules. Milk thistle is one of the few herbs that are very effective in capsule form, and almost all commercially available brands are good quality. The best strategy is to take 2 capsules with a big glass of water before you start drinking, another 2 before bed, and 2 more in the morning. Sometimes this will prevent you from getting a hangover at all!

TAKE-IT-EASY NEXT DAY INFUSION

Makes about 3¼ cups dried herb mix (enough for 20 to 28 quarts of tea)
This gentle tea calms the most common hangover symptoms and helps with rehydration to boot. Best to mix it up before the big party, so it'll be ready when you need it. Drink a quart or more, slowly, over the course of the day.

½ cup dried betony leaf and flower
½ cup dried plantain leaf
½ cup dried calendula flower
½ cup dried chamomile flower
⅓ cup dried linden leaf and flower

⅓ cup dried marshmallow leaf
⅓ cup dried self-heal leaf and flower
1 tablespoon dried licorice root
1 tablespoon dried ginger
¼ cup dried St. John's wort leaf and flower

1.In a medium bowl, mix together all the herbs. Store in an airtight container.
2.Make a hot infusion: Prepare a kettle of boiling water. Measure 2 to 3 tablespoons of herbs per quart of water and place in a mason jar or French press. Pour in the boiling water, cover, and steep for 20 minutes or until cool enough to drink.

TIP: Omit the St. John's wort if you are concurrently taking pharmaceuticals.

NO~FUSS HANGOVER TEA

1 teaspoon ripe barberry berries
1 teaspoon Oregon grape root
2 cups boiling water

1. Combine the herbs in a nonmetallic container and cover with the boiling water; steep for 30 minutes; cool and strain.
2. Take up to one cup a day, diluted in plenty of cool water.

QUICK~ACTING HANGOVER TEA

1 teaspoon bayberry root
1 teaspoon dried goldenseal root
1 teaspoon Oregon grape root
2 cups boiling water

1. Combine the herbs in a nonmetallic container and cover with the boiling water; steep for 30 minutes; strain.
2. Place a tablespoon of the mixture in an 8-ounce glass of water.
3. Drink several glasses throughout the day.

SPICY HANGOVER TEA

1 teaspoon catnip leaves
1 teaspoon peppermint leaves

1 teaspoon dried chaparral leaves
2 cups boiling water

1. Combine the herbs in a nonmetallic container and cover with the boiling water; steep for 20 to 30 minutes; strain.
2. Drink half a cup at a time, up to two cups a day.

Headache

Headaches are very common and can be dull and steady, stabbing, gnawing, or throbbing. There are many kinds of headaches with many different causes. Sometimes tension, fatigue, or stress can cause a headache. Problems with the eyes, ears, nose, throat, or teeth can bring on a headache, as can allergies, injuries, infection, tumors, and any number of diseases. Headaches are also big business. In fact, Americans spend in excess of $1 billion each year buying medicines to help combat headaches. Most people take nonsteroidal anti-inflammatory drugs (NSAIDs) such as aspirin, ibuprofen, or indomethacin, or even stronger painkillers. But these drugs have unwanted, and sometimes serious, side effects, including ulcers and an increased tendency to bleeding. Herbs can offer a safer alternative.

Relevant tissue states: heat or cold, damp or dry, tense or lax
Relevant herbal actions: anodyne, anti-inflammatory, astringent, circulatory stimulant, relaxant

Herbal Allies

- Betony leaf and flower
- Catnip
- Chamomile flower
- Feverfew
- Peppermint
- Pleurisy root
- White Willow
- Wintergreen
- Ginger
- Linden leaf and flower
- Marshmallow
- Meadowsweet flower
- Sage leaf
- Tulsi leaf
- Wild lettuce

Headaches arise from a variety of imbalances. Some are simple one-off causes—dehydration, sleep debt, dietary excesses, alcohol, caffeine, medications. For those, you want quick pain relief while you supply what's missing or simply wait for the body to recover. (When unsure of where to start, turn to betony.)

For long-term relief, it's important to identify your individual triggers, as well as the underlying patterns that contribute to your pain; this takes some experimentation. The following herbal remedies are designed to address the most common types of headaches we see, but try different combinations of herbs to refine the remedy and make it as personal as possible. If you have recurrent headaches and find this helps, drink a quart or more every day as a preventive.

COOLING HEADACHE TEA

Makes 3¼ cups dried herb mix (enough for 22 to 28 quarts of tea)

If a headache makes you turn red-faced, and the pain feels hot, sharp, and very sensitive to the touch, this is for you. This kind of headache often results from tension, stress or anxiety, sinus congestion, or direct nerve pain. These herbs cool, relax (be aware the wild lettuce may make you sleepy), and drain.

1 cup dried betony leaf and flower
1 cup dried meadowsweet flower
½ cup dried linden leaf and flower
½ cup dried marshmallow leaf
¼ cup dried wild lettuce leaf and stalk

1.In a medium bowl, mix together all the herbs. Store in an airtight container.
2.Make a hot infusion: Prepare a kettle of boiling water. Measure 2 to 3 tablespoons of herbs per quart of water and place in a mason jar or French press. Pour in the boiling water, cover, and steep for 30 to 40 minutes. Drink warm or cool. One cup of this tea should begin to give some relief.

WARMING HEADACHE TEA

Makes 3¼ cups dried herb mix (enough for 22 to 28 quarts of tea)

If, when your headaches strike, you have a pale face and the pain feels cold, dull, and broad, try this blend. This type of headache is often caused by hypothyroidism, liver congestion, and circulatory stagnation. These herbs warm, gently astringe, and improve circulation. (If caffeine usually works as a headache remedy for you, try this.) If you have recurrent headaches and find this helps, drink a quart or more every day as a preventive.

1 cup dried betony leaf and flower
1 cup dried tulsi leaf
½ cup dried chamomile flower
½ cup dried sage leaf
¼ cup dried ginger

1.In a medium bowl, mix together all the herbs. Store in an airtight container.
2.Make a hot infusion: Prepare a kettle of boiling water. Measure 2 to 3 tablespoons of herbs per quart of water and place in a mason jar or French press. Pour in the boiling water, cover, and steep for 30 to 40 minutes. Drink warm to hot. One cup of this tea should begin to give some relief.

PEPPERY HEADACHE TEA

1 teaspoon feverfew leaves
1 teaspoon peppermint leaves

1 cup boiling water
Honey

1. Combine the above herbs in a nonmetallic container and cover with the boiling water; steep for 30 minutes; strain.
2. Add honey to taste. Take a tablespoon at a time, up to one cup a day.

SOOTHING HEADACHE TEA

1 teaspoon catnip leaves
2 teaspoons feverfew leaves
1 to 2 cups boiling water

1. Combine the catnip and the feverfew in a glass container.
2. Pour one to two cups of boiling water over the herbs; steep for 30 minutes; strain.
3. Take up to one cup a day, a tablespoon at a time.

HEARTBURN/REFLUX/GERD

Heartburn is burning stomach pain that can spread up into your throat. Heartburn occurs when hydrochloric acid from your stomach backs up into the esophagus. This condition can result if you gulp your food or drink too much caffeine or alcohol. It can also occur if you eat while stressed or eat certain foods (such as spicy or fatty foods). Antacids are commonly taken for heartburn, but herbs can be just as effective.

Note: If you suffer from heartburn, avoid peppermint. Although it is helpful in treating indigestion and other stomach problems, it can relax the esophageal sphincter and actually increase the tendency toward heartburn.

Relevant tissue states: heat (inflammation), laxity
Relevant herbal actions: bitter, carminative, demulcent, vulnerary

Herbal Allies

- Barberry
- Bayberry
- Catnip leaf and flower
- Chamomile flower
- Chaparral
- Coriander
- Dandelion root
- Fennel seed
- Ginger

- Hops
- Kelp
- Licorice root
- Linden leaf and flower
- Marshmallow
- Meadowsweet flower
- Oregon grape
- Self-heal leaf and flower
- St. John's wort leaf and flower
- Yellow Dock

Contrary to what you might expect, heartburn is most often caused by low levels of stomach acid. When stomach acid is low, it causes a chain of problems in the digestive system that ultimately increase upward-moving pressure in the abdomen. This weakens the "trapdoor" between the stomach and the esophagus—when that's compromised, acid is more likely to splash up through and irritate the unprotected tissue there.

Reducing stomach acid production (with antacids or acid-blocking pharmaceuticals) temporarily relieves pain, but makes the underlying problem worse. To address heartburn, first we have to heal existing damage in the esophagus or stomach (inflammation and ulcers). Then we can work to restore normal acid levels to prevent recurrence.

That stomach-esophagus "trapdoor" (the lower esophageal sphincter, LES) can also be compromised by poor alignment and stress. When in a state of stress, saliva production decreases and digestive movement is inhibited. A rest-and-digest state of mind is required to retain the proper resting tone of the LES. This starts by being present with your food—slow down, chew thoroughly, take your time.

MARSHMALLOW INFUSION

Makes 1 quart

If you have active heartburn, the first thing you need is a good cold infusion of marshmallow root. Keep this on hand for when there's an attack and to heal the damaged tissue in the esophagus. When heartburn happens, just sip on this slowly and you'll feel relief in no time.

2 to 4 tablespoons dried marshmallow root

In a quart-size mason jar, combine the marshmallow with enough cold or room-temperature water to fill the jar. Cover and steep for 4 to 8 hours. Keep refrigerated, where each batch will last for 2 to 3 days.

PREVENTIVE BITTER TINCTURE

Makes 3½ fluid ounces (30 to 60 doses)

To restore normal stomach acid levels and reduce the conditions for heartburn to develop, take these drops before every meal.

1 fluid ounce tincture of dandelion root
½ fluid ounce tincture of catnip
½ fluid ounce tincture of chamomile
⅓ fluid ounce tincture of fennel
⅓ fluid ounce tincture of meadowsweet
⅓ fluid ounce tincture of self-heal
½ fluid ounce tincture of St. John's wort (see Tip)

1. In a small bottle, combine the tinctures. Cap the bottle and label it.
2. Take ½ to 1 dropperful 10 minutes before eating.

TIP: Omit the St. John's wort if you are concurrently taking pharmaceuticals.

QUICK-ACTING HEARTBURN TEA

1 teaspoon dried angelica root
1 teaspoon crushed juniper berries
1 cup boiling water

1. Combine the herbs in a nonmetallic container and cover with the boiling water; steep for 20 to 30 minutes; strain.
2. Take a tablespoon at a time, as needed.

SOOTHING HEARTBURN TEA

1 teaspoon catnip leaves
1 teaspoon oxeye daisy herb
1 cup boiling water

1. Combine the herbs in a non-metallic container and cover with the boiling water; steep for 30 minutes; strain.
2. Take a tablespoon at a time, as needed.

Hypertension

The list of circulatory disorders is almost endless and includes heart disease, strokes, hypertension, and atherosclerosis, to name a few. These and other circulatory conditions are the number-one cause of death in this country, killing nearly one million Americans every year.

As we age, our body's ability to keep a proper equilibrium between blood clotting and blood liquefaction begins to go awry. On the one hand, blood must clot if we are to keep from bleeding to death, yet, on the other hand, it must be free flowing and liquid in order to travel easily through the body's blood vessels. The older we get, the "stickier" our blood gets, and our blood's ability to flow diminishes. When this occurs, the stage is set for blood clots, clogged arteries, strokes, and heart attacks.

Relevant tissue states: heat, tension
Relevant herbal actions: hypotensive, nervine, relaxant, sedative

Herbal Allies

- Black Cohosh
- Black Currant
- Burdock
- Cayenne
- Dandelion
- Garlic
- Ginger
- Gingko Biloba
- Ginseng
- Goldenseal
- Gotu Kola
- Kelp
- Linden leaf and flower
- Marshmallow
- Raspberry
- Rose
- Slippery Elm
- Yarrow leaf and flower

Occasional high blood pressure is normal—it's a part of the natural response to stressful situations. Over time, though, high blood pressure can cause or worsen other cardiovascular problems. Herbs offer a nice suite of actions to reduce high blood pressure, often by addressing root causes rather than merely acting symptomatically.

It's worth noting that high blood pressure isn't always bad: New information indicates that hypertension that develops in the elder years may actually help reduce the risk of dementia.

SOFTHEARTED TEA

Makes 2 cups dried herb mix (enough for 12 to 16 quarts of tea)

Reducing stress makes a big difference, so herbs that can relax the mind while soothing the physical heart are ideal. For those with very dry constitutions, prepare this as a cold infusion instead. Drink a quart or more every day.

1 cup dried linden leaf and flower

½ cup dried marshmallow leaf
½ cup dried rose petals

1.In a small bowl, mix together all the herbs. Store in an airtight container.
2.Make a hot infusion: Prepare a kettle of boiling water. Measure 2 to 3 tablespoons of herbs per quart of water and place in a mason jar or French press. Pour in the boiling water, cover, and steep for 20 minutes or until cool enough to drink.

FREE~FLOWING CIRCULATION TEA

1 teaspoon burdock root
1 teaspoon goldenseal root
1 teaspoon cayenne
2 teaspoons slippery elm bark
2 slices ginger root
3 cups boiling water

1. Combine the above herbs in a nonmetallic container, and pour the boiling water over them. Steep for 30 minutes, cool, and strain.
2. Take up to one cup a day, two tablespoons at a time.

ANTI~CONGESTIVE TEA

2 teaspoons black cohosh root
4 teaspoons ginkgo biloba leaves
2 cups boiling water

1. Combine the above herbs in a nonmetallic container, and pour the boiling water over them. Soak for 30 minutes, cool, and strain.
2. Take two to three tablespoons at a time, up to six times a day.

ARTERIOSCLEROSIS PREVENTIVE TEA

2 to 3 ginger slices
2 teaspoons Ginkgo biloba leaves
1 teaspoon ginseng leaves
2 cups boiling water

1. Combine the herbs in a nonmetallic container and cover with the boiling water.

2. Steep for 30 minutes, cool, and strain.
3. Take up to half a cup per day.

Indigestion/Dyspepsia

Indigestion refers to any gastrointestinal disturbance, such as an upset stomach. Indigestion can occur if you eat too fast, eat too much, eat while emotionally upset, or, for some people, eat the wrong foods. Caffeine, high-fiber foods, alcohol, and carbonated drinks are often indigestion culprits. Sometimes allergies can cause indigestion. Indigestion can be a symptom of a number of diseases, including pancreatitis, ulcers, gastritis, and cholecystis. Often, however, there is no known cause for indigestion.

Relevant tissue states: cold (stagnation), tension
Relevant herbal actions: bitter, carminative, relaxant

Herbal Allies

- Angelica
- Barberry
- Bayberry
- Blue Cohosh
- Catnip leaf and flower
- Chamomile flower
- Coneflower
- Dandelion root
- Echinacea
- Fennel seed
- Ginger
- Licorice root
- Oregon Grape
- Peppermint leaf
- Sage leaf

If you're having chronic digestive discomforts, take a hard look at your diet to see if you have any food sensitivities. Lucky for you, though, indigestion is a problem for which herbal quick fixes are ready at hand—read on for two simple, portable solutions.

PRE~EMPTIVE BITTER TINCTURE

Makes 4 fluid ounces (60 to 120 doses)

Indigestion often means just that—incomplete digestion. This formula stimulates all your digestive fluids—saliva, stomach acid, bile, and pancreatic enzymes—so digestion is as thorough and complete as possible.

1 fluid ounce tincture of dandelion root
1 fluid ounce tincture of sage
1 fluid ounce tincture of catnip
1 fluid ounce tincture of chamomile

1. In a small bottle, combine the tinctures. Cap the bottle and label it.
2. Take 1 to 2 drops 10 minutes before eating.

CARMINATIVE TINCTURE

Makes 4 fluid ounces (60 to 120 doses)

This formula warms the body's core, stimulating your digestive organs and keeping the bowels from getting sluggish. If peppermint isn't your style, substitute angelica.

1½ fluid ounces tincture of ginger
1 fluid ounce tincture of fennel
1 fluid ounce tincture of peppermint (see headnote)
½ fluid ounce tincture of licorice

1. In a small bottle, combine the tinctures. Cap the bottle and label it.
2. Take 1 to 2 drops after each meal, or whenever your guts feel uncomfortably stuck.

DIGESTIVE TEA

1 teaspoon blue cohosh root
1 teaspoon coneflower root
1 cup boiling water

1. Combine the above herbs in a glass container.
2. Pour the boiling water over the herbs; steep for 30 minutes; cool and strain.
3. Take as needed, up to one cup a day.

STRONG DIGESTIVE TEA

1 teaspoon angelica root
1 teaspoon grated ginger root
2 teaspoons chamomile flowers
2 teaspoons peppermint leaves
1 cup boiling water

1. Combine the above ingredients in a container.
2. Take one tablespoon of the herb mixture and place in the boiling water; steep for 30 minutes; cool and strain.
3. Take as needed, up to two cups a day.

QUICK~ACTING DIGESTIVE TEA

1 teaspoon licorice root
1 teaspoon peppermint leaves
2 cups boiling water

1. Combine the above herbs in a nonmetallic container and cover with the boiling water; steep for 15 to 20 minutes; strain.
2. Take as needed, up to one cup a day.

Insomnia

Insomnia is any difficulty in sleeping. Some people find it difficult to fall asleep, while others can fall asleep easily but don't stay asleep. Nearly one-fourth of all Americans have an occasional problem sleeping, but some people (as much as 10 percent of the American population) suffer from chronic insomnia. Insomnia can occur for a number of reasons, including stress and nervous tension, excessive intake of caffeinated drinks, and irregular sleeping habits.

Insomnia can lead to fatigue and an inability to function at an optimal energy level during the day. Irritability, daytime drowsiness, and memory impairment often affect those suffering from insomnia.

Relevant tissue states: heat (agitation), tension
Relevant herbal actions: hypnotic, relaxant, sedative

Herbal Allies

- Ashwagandha root
- Betony leaf and flower
- Catnip leaf and flower
- Chamomile flower
- Hops
- Linden leaf and flower
- Passionflower
- Rose
- Valerian
- Wild lettuce

Wild animals don't have insomnia. Hikers in the wilds don't either, actually. According to a 2013 study in the journal Current Biology, just a few days in an outdoor environment, with no artificial light exposure, is enough to reestablish normal circadian rhythms—even in people who are habitual "night owls" in their city lives. This tracks with a large and growing body of evidence that indicates that our electrically lit environments are directly responsible for most sleep disturbances we experience.

Reducing evening exposure to bright lights—including TV, computer, and smartphone screens—is one of the most important steps you can take to fight insomnia. Dimming lights and avoiding screens for at least an hour before bed, and taking the herbal remedies offered here, are sure ways to improve both the quantity and quality of your sleep.

END-OF-THE-DAY ELIXIR

Makes 4 fluid ounces (60 to 120 doses)

This blend of relaxants and gentle sedatives doesn't force sleep but helps relieve the tension, anxiety, and distraction that make it difficult to transition into sleep. This formula (and any herbs taken to aid in sleep) is best taken in "pulse doses," which is much more effective than taking the total dose all at once right at bedtime. It gives the herbs time to start working in your system and emphasizes to the body that it's time to transition into sleep.

1 fluid ounce tincture of chamomile

1 fluid ounce tincture of betony
¾ fluid ounce tincture of ashwagandha
½ fluid ounce tincture of catnip
½ fluid ounce tincture of linden
¼ fluid ounce honey (plain or rose petal–infused)

1.In a small bottle, combine the tinctures and honey. Cap the bottle and label it.
2.One hour before bedtime, take 1 to 2 drops.
3.Thirty minutes before bedtime, take another 1 to 2 drops.
4.At bedtime, take the final 1 to 2 drops.

SLEEP! FORMULA

Makes 4 fluid ounces (60 to 120 doses)

For this formula, we recruit wild lettuce, the strongest hypnotic (sleep-inducing) herb in this book. This is especially helpful if part of what's keeping you up at night is physical pain, as wild lettuce also has a pain-relieving effect. This formula, like End-of-the-Day Elixir, is best taken in "pulse doses."

2 fluid ounces tincture of wild lettuce
1 fluid ounce tincture of betony
½ fluid ounce tincture of chamomile
½ fluid ounce tincture of linden

1.In a small bottle, combine the tinctures. Cap the bottle and label it.
2.One hour before bedtime, take 1 to 2 drops.
3.Thirty minutes before bedtime, take another 1 to 2 drops.
4.At bedtime, take the final 1 to 2 drops.

INSOMNIA RELIEF TEA

1 teaspoon chamomile flowers
1 teaspoon hops
1 teaspoon valerian root
1 cup boiling water

1. Combine the above herbs.
2. Take one tablespoon of the mixture and cover with the boiling water; let steep for 30 minutes; strain.
3. Drink warm, as needed, half a cup at a time.

SWEET DREAMS TEA

2 teaspoons catnip leaves
1 teaspoon hops
2 teaspoons chamomile flower
2 teaspoons passionflower
1 cup boiling water

1. Combine the above herbs in a glass container; cover with the boiling water; steep for 30 minutes; cool and strain.
2. Take one hour before bedtime.

Menstrual cycle irregularities

The irregularities include various disruptions of the menstrual cycle. Each is addressed slightly differently, but a few overarching actions emerge that help with all of them: nourishing the body, improving circulation, and stimulating the liver and kidneys to clear away used-up hormones.

Delayed or absent menses may be due to a lack of adequate nourishment, especially protein, or to disruptions in hormone levels. (Sometimes these share a cause. A high-sugar diet is nutrient-poor, and the havoc it wreaks on blood sugar levels has a cascade effect that disrupts hormone balance. Stress makes us tend to eat gratifying but poor-quality food, and excessive stress-response hormones interfere with the normal actions of estrogen and progesterone.)

Irregular cycles, with no predictable pattern, may also be due to poor nourishment, liver stagnation or strain, or an irregular lifestyle—especially erratic sleep habits. The daily cycle shapes the monthly cycle, like small and large gears interlocking in a watch.

Overheavy bleeding generally comes from hormones not clearing efficiently at the liver, though it may also be connected with the development of fibroids or polyps. If heavy bleeding persists, seek medical attention.

Finally, let's talk about the most common menstrual ailment: dysmenorrhea, or menstrual pain, which usually begins just before menstruation, may occur in the lower abdomen or the lower back (and sometimes even into the thighs). Other accompanying symptoms may include nausea, vomiting, headache, and either constipation or diarrhea. This condition affects more than half of all women.

There are two types of dysmenorrhea, primary and secondary. In primary dysmenorrhea, there is no underlying pain causing the disorder. It is thought that the pain occurs when uterine contractions reduce blood supply to the uterus. This may occur if the uterus is in the wrong position, if the cervical opening is narrow, and due to lack of exercise.

Secondary dysmenorrhea is when the pain is caused by some gynecological disorder, such as endometriosis (when the endometrium, the tissue that lines the uterus, abnormally grows on surfaces of other structures in the abdominal cavity), adenomyosis (in-growth of the endometrium into the uterine musculature), lesions, inflammation of the fallopian tubes, or uterine fibroids. Uterine fibroids are tumors of the uterus that are not usually cancerous. Also known as myomas, these masses occur in nearly one-quarter of all women by the age of forty. Some women with uterine fibroids may have no symptoms. However, if symptoms are present they include increased frequency of urination, a bloated feeling, pressure, pain, and abnormal bleeding.

Relevant tissue states: cold (stagnation), laxity
Relevant herbal actions: astringent, carminative, circulatory stimulant, emmenagogue, nutritive, rubefacient

- Angelica
- Ashwagandha root
- Betony leaf and flower
- Black Cohosh
- Blue Vervain
- Chamomile flower
- Crampbark
- Dandelion leaf
- Elecampane
- Feverfew
- Ginger
- Goldenrod leaf and flower
- Kelp
- Marigold
- Milk thistle seed
- Nettle leaf
- Passionflower
- Peppermint
- Pulsatilla
- Raspberry
- Sage leaf
- Self-heal leaf and flower
- St. John's Wort
- Tulsi leaf

STEADY CYCLE TEA

Makes 3½ cups dried herb mix (enough for 20 to 28 quarts of tea)

These herbs provide substantial nourishment and a bit of gentle kidney, lymphatic, and endocrine stimulation. Long-term use of a formula like this has been the major factor in improvement for a great many of our clients with menstrual irregularities of all types. Add ginger if you run cold, betony if you're frequently anxious, and peppermint for taste (if you like it). Drink a quart or more every day.

1 cup dried nettle leaf
1 cup dried dandelion leaf
½ cup dried goldenrod leaf and flower
½ cup dried self-heal leaf and flower
¼ cup dried tulsi leaf
¼ cup dried kelp

1.In a small bowl, mix together all the herbs. Store in an airtight container.
2.Make a long infusion: Prepare a kettle of boiling water. Measure 2 to 3 tablespoons of herbs per quart of water and place in a mason jar or French press. Pour in the boiling water, cover, and steep for 8 hours or overnight.

BLEED ON! TEA

Makes 3 cups dried herb mix (enough for 20 to 26 quarts of tea)

To bring on menstruation, drink this tea for 3 days to 1 week prior to the expected start of your next period. Drink this tea very hot for best results. Reheat as necessary and drink a quart or more over the course of the day. For a stronger effect, take a drop of angelica tincture together with each cup of tea.

1 cup dried chamomile flower
1 cup dried tulsi leaf
⅓ cup dried goldenrod leaf and flower
⅓ cup dried ginger
⅓ cup dried angelica root

1. In a small bowl, mix together all the herbs. Store in an airtight container.
2. Make a hot infusion: Prepare a kettle of boiling water. Measure 2 to 3 tablespoons of herbs per quart of water and place in a mason jar or French press. Pour in the boiling water, cover, and steep for 20 minutes or until cool enough to drink.

DAILY SOOTHING MENSTRUAL TEA

2 teaspoons black haw root or bark
2 teaspoons passionflower
2 cups cold water

1. Combine the above herbs in a pan and cover with the cold water; soak overnight; strain.
2. Take half a cup, up to four times daily.

DYSMENORRHEA TEA

2 teaspoons black cohosh root
1 teaspoon crampbark
1 teaspoon black haw root or bark
1 teaspoon pulsatilla
2 cups water

1. Combine the above herbs in a pan and cover with the water; bring to a boil and boil for 10 minutes; cool and strain.
2. Take half a cup, up to four times a day.

CRAMP RELIEF TEA

1 teaspoon St. John's wort leaves
1 teaspoon raspberry leaves
1 cup boiling water

1. Combine the herbs in a glass container and cover with the boiling water; steep for 15 minutes; strain.
2. Drink as needed to relieve cramps.

Nausea and Vomiting

Nausea is an unpleasant feeling that you are about to vomit. It is often accompanied by excess salivation and sometimes stomach cramping. A number of diseases and conditions can cause nausea, including food poisoning (and other bacterial infections), viral infections, overeating or overdrinking, gallstones, pancreatitis, and cancer. It can also occur because of motion sickness, headache, or pregnancy. Sometimes unpleasant smells or tastes, and even emotional anxiety, can bring on nausea.

Relevant tissue states: heat (agitation), tension (spasm)
Relevant herbal actions: antiemetic, carminative, relaxant

Herbal Allies

- Bayberry
- Bee Balm
- Catnip leaf and flower
- Chamomile flower
- Chaparral
- Fennel seed
- Ginger
- Horehound
- Oregon Grape
- Peppermint leaf
- Yerba mansa

One way or another, nausea almost always comes from food—a sensitivity, some indigestion, various potential infections. Especially if nausea happens frequently, look closely at your diet—keeping a journal can be helpful—to identify any patterns that occur around its appearance. Maybe when you eat on the run, or eat wheat products, or have really fiery spices—whatever it is for you, the only way to identify it is to pay attention in an organized way.

After a bout of vomiting, some warm, slightly weak Calming Tea can be the easiest thing to drink for quite some time. Then slowly reintroduce broth, then soup, then stew . . . gradually progressing from food prepared to be very warm and moist to food that is more cool and dry, like salad.

Both of the following formulas are also excellent for morning sickness. If you feel you can't get anything down at all, just one drop of ginger tincture all by itself on the tongue can be helpful, or even just smelling strong ginger tea.

CALMING TEA

Makes 3¼ cups dried herb mix (enough for 20 to 26 quarts of tea)

For most cases of nausea, this combination of the best herbal antiemetics should help very quickly. If you know you prefer (or dislike) the flavor of one of these ingredients, feel free to adjust its proportion. This also helps as a preventive—if prone to nausea, drink a quart or more every day.

1 cup dried catnip leaf and flower
1 cup dried chamomile flower
½ cup dried peppermint leaf
½ cup fennel seed
¼ cup dried ginger

1. In a medium bowl, mix together all the herbs. Store in an airtight container.
2. Make a hot infusion: Prepare a kettle of boiling water. Measure 2 to 3 tablespoons of herbs per quart of water and place in a mason jar or French press. Pour in the boiling water, cover, and steep for 20 minutes or until cool enough to drink.
3. Drink a cupful, slowly, in small sips. If the nausea is very severe, just sit for a while and inhale the scent rising off the hot tea.

GINGER EMERGENCY FORMULA

Makes 5 fluid ounces (60 to 120 doses)

This mixture of tinctures is one to keep in your herbal first aid kit at all times. You never know when nausea will strike, and a quick herbal relief will be very welcome. Make this with ginger-infused honey if you have the time to prepare that in advance.

2 fluid ounces tincture of ginger
1 fluid ounce tincture of catnip
1 fluid ounce tincture of chamomile
1 fluid ounce honey

1. In a small bottle, combine all the ingredients. Cap the bottle and label it.
2. Take 1 to 2 droppersful every 20 minutes until relief occurs.

ANTIEMETIC TEA

1 teaspoon grated ginger root
1 teaspoon yerba mansa root
1 teaspoon peppermint leaves
2 cups boiling water

1. Combine the above herbs in a nonmetallic container and cover with the boiling water; steep for 30 minutes; cool and strain.

2. Take as needed, a tablespoon at a time, up to two cups a day.

NAUSEA-SOOTHING TEA

1 teaspoon catnip leaves
1 teaspoon chamomile flowers
1 cup boiling water

1. Combine the above ingredients in a nonmetallic container and cover with the boiling water; steep for 20 to 30 minutes; cool and strain.

2. Take as needed.

Rash

A skin rash is a temporary eruption on the skin that usually looks like small red or pink bumps. It may or may not itch. There may be scaly, round, or oval patches on the skin. A rash is usually a symptom of some other condition and can indicate a disease such as measles or chickenpox, an insect bite, an allergic reaction, a nutritional deficiency, or even dry skin.

Relevant tissue states: heat (inflammation), dryness or dampness, laxity
Relevant herbal actions: anti-inflammatory, astringent, demulcent

Herbal Allies

- Burdock
- Calendula flower
- Comfrey
- Echinacea
- Evening Primrose
- Goldenseal
- Kelp
- Licorice root
- Marshmallow
- Oregon grape
- Plantain leaf
- Rose
- Self-heal leaf and flower
- Slippery Elm
- St. John's wort leaf and flower
- Strawberry
- Uva-ursi leaf
- White oak
- Yarrow leaf and flower
- Yellow Dock

A sudden appearance of a rash generally means you've come into contact with some kind of irritant—an irritating plant, a toxic chemical, or perhaps an insect bite or sting. Wash the area well with soap and water. Then apply insights from basic herbal energetics: If the rash is dry, use moistening herbs and preparations; if it's damp and oozy, use drying agents.

If there doesn't seem to have been any contact with an irritating plant, chemical, or other direct trigger, the rash may be an external reflection of an internal imbalance. Allergies can cause this, of course, as well as overworked internal detoxification systems.

DRY RASH SALVE

Makes 9 ounces (60-day supply)

Salves are emollient due to their oil and wax content, especially when they have a moisturizing oil, like olive oil, as the base. In this simple formula, the herbs' healing and anti-inflammatory effects enhance the emollient effect.

3 fluid ounces calendula-infused oil
3 fluid ounces plantain-infused oil
2 fluid ounces licorice-infused oil
1 ounce beeswax, plus more as needed

1.Prepare a salve as usual (see here for complete instructions).
2.Gently apply a thin layer to the affected area at least twice a day.

WEEPY RASH POULTICE

Makes 4½ cups dried herb mix (enough for 12 to 18 poultices)

Contact with poison ivy and similar plants often produces a rash with fluid-filled blisters. These call for astringents, and those are best delivered in a water extract—a poultice or compress.
Learn to identify the plants that cause contact rash in your area! Poison ivy, poison oak, and poison sumac all grow in the US. Check out poison-ivy.org for great pictures and details about how to make a positive identification, as well as how to tell them apart from benign look-alike plants.

1 cup dried calendula flower
1 cup dried rose petals
1 cup dried self-heal leaf and flower
½ cup dried St. John's wort leaf and flower
½ cup dried uva-ursi leaf
½ cup dried yarrow leaf and flower
Boiling water, to make the poultice

1.In a large bowl, mix together all the herbs. Store in an airtight container.
2.Measure 4 to 6 tablespoons of the herb mixture and place in a heat-proof dish.
3.Pour just enough boiling water over the herbs to get them fully saturated—not so much that they're swimming. Let the herbs soak for 5 minutes.
4.Apply the mass of herbs, warm and wet, to the affected area. Cover with a cloth. Keep in place for 5 to 10 minutes, then gently pat dry.
5.Repeat 1 to 3 times per day.

TIP: If you don't have these herbs on hand, plain green or black tea bags will do the trick! Just get them warm and wet, apply them over the rash, and let them sit in place for 20 minutes.

SKIN~SOOTHING TEA

1 teaspoon burdock root
1 teaspoon Oregon grape root
1 teaspoon echinacea root
1 teaspoon yellow dock root
2 cups water

1. Combine the above herbs in a pan and cover with the water. Bring to a boil; reduce heat and simmer for 10 to 15 minutes; cool and strain.

2. Take a tablespoon at a time, up to half a cup a day.

RASH WASH

1 teaspoon comfrey root
1 teaspoon white oak leaves or bark
1 teaspoon slippery elm bark
2 cups water

1. Place the herbs in a container and cover with the water; bring to a boil and boil for 20 to 30 minutes; cool and strain.
2. Use as a topical wash, as needed.

Sinusitis/Stuffy Nose

Sinusitis is an inflammation of the sinuses, marked by sinus congestion, headache, and pain around the eyes or cheeks. There may be a nasal discharge, fatigue, cough, fever, earache, and an increased susceptibility to nasal infections.

Sinusitis can be caused by allergies, bacterial or fungal infections, and viral infections (such as the common cold). However, nasal injury, a deviated septum (the separator between the two nasal passages), a swollen conchae (the spiral air warmers in the nose), nasal polyps, or narrow sinuses can also cause sinusitis, as can cigarette smoke, dusty or dry air, or even infected tonsils or teeth.

Relevant tissue states: heat (inflammation), laxity (mucous membranes)
Relevant herbal actions: antifungal, anti-inflammatory, antimicrobial, astringent, decongestant, demulcent

Herbal Allies

- Bayberry
- Black Elder
- Calendula flower
- Echinacea
- Garlic
- Ginger
- Gingko Biloba
- Ginseng
- Goldenrod leaf and flower
- Goldenseal
- Licorice
- Pau D'Arco
- Pine
- Rose
- Slippery Elm
- Valerian
- White Willow
- Wild Indigo
- Witch Hazel
- Marshmallow
- Sage leaf
- Thyme leaf
- Uva-ursi leaf
- Yerba mansa

Runny nose is a vital response to a cold or the flu! Believe it or not, mucus is full of antibodies. Drying it up with pharmaceutical decongestants makes the tissue more susceptible to infection. Keeping mucous membranes at a happy medium—not too dry, not too drippy—helps shorten the illness and prevent complications.

If not connected to a full respiratory infection, or if chronic or recurrent, the cause of symptoms is likely a complex of bacterial, fungal, and viral components. (This is why it can persist even after multiple rounds of antibiotics.) Antimicrobial herbs are less specific than antibiotic drugs, which is a benefit in this case, meaning that they can counteract a variety of pathogens and compromised states simultaneously.

Grating fresh horseradish and breathing its fumes, or eating prepared horseradish or wasabi, is a great way to clear the sinuses. If you've been blowing your nose a lot and the skin is irritated, some soft, simple salve or lanolin is very soothing.

SINUS~CLEARING STEAM BATH

Makes 2 cups dried herb mix (enough for 4 to 8 steams)

Steaming is a universal treatment across cultures for any respiratory system troubles, including those related to the sinuses. The combination of hot steam and the evaporating volatile oils from the herbs makes it very difficult for pathogens to survive and stimulates immune response in the mucous membranes.

1 cup dried pine needles
½ cup dried sage leaf
½ cup dried thyme leaf
½ gallon water
5 garlic cloves, chopped, per steam (optional)

1. In a small bowl, mix the pine, sage, and thyme. Store in an airtight container.
2. Make and execute an herbal steam: In a medium pot over high heat, boil the water.
3. Place the pot on a heat-proof surface, someplace where you can sit near it, and make a tent with a blanket or towel.
4. Add ¼ to ½ cup of the herb mixture to the water, along with the garlic (if using).
5. Position your face over the steam and remain there for 5 to 20 minutes. (Bring a handkerchief, your nose will run as your sinuses clear!)
6. Repeat 2 to 3 times per day.

TIP: Similar microbe-clearing benefits can be gained by working with aromatic herbs as incense or a smudge stick (a tightly wrapped bundle of leaves, lit on one end to produce medicinal smoke). A study by Nautiyal et al. in the Journal of Ethnopharmacology found that "[when] using medicinal smoke[,] it is possible to completely eliminate diverse plant and human pathogenic bacteria of the air within confined space." Conifer trees like pine are particularly apt for this.

SINUS~RELIEVING TEA

1 teaspoon echinacea root
1 teaspoon yerba mansa root
1 teaspoon goldenseal root
1 cup boiling water

1. Combine the above herbs.
2. Take two teaspoons of the mixture and cover with the boiling water; steep for 20 to 30 minutes; strain.
3. Take warm, up to one cup per day, as needed.

MUCUS~FREEING TEA

1 teaspoon bayberry root
1 teaspoon white willow bark
2 cups boiling water

1. Combine the above herbs and cover with the boiling water; steep for 15 minutes.
2. Take warm, up to two cups a day.

Sore Throat

Usually, a sore throat is a minor problem that takes care of itself with time. Although we may not always be able to identify the cause of a sore throat, it most often occurs because of viral infections such as the flu or a common cold. It can also occur because of exposure to irritants such as dust or smoke, from allergies, or even from talking or yelling too loudly. A sore throat may make swallowing difficult and may lead to a hoarse voice.

Relevant tissue states: heat (inflammation), dryness or dampness
Relevant herbal actions: anti-inflammatory, antimicrobial, astringent, demulcent, mucous membrane tonic

Herbal Allies

- Balsam Fir
- Bayberry
- Black Elder
- Blue Vervain
- Canadian Fleabane
- Cayenne
- Cinnamon bark
- Coltsfoot
- Comfrey
- Echinacea
- Ginger
- Goldenrod leaf and flower
- Indian Root
- Licorice root
- Marshmallow
- Osha Root
- Sage leaf
- Self-heal leaf and flower
- Seneca Snakeroot
- Slippery Elm
- Sumac
- Wild Cherry
- Witch Hazel
- Yerba sante

Sore throats are generally due to infection, whether that's a simple cold, the flu, or strep throat. When choosing remedies, it is helpful to differentiate between the hot, inflamed, dry sore throat and the cold, wet sore throat induced by post-nasal drip. Use extra demulcents for the former and astringent mucous membrane tonics for the latter. See also Cold and Flu and Immune Support.

SORE THROAT TEA

Makes 2 cups dried herb mix (enough for 12 to 16 quarts of tea)

If you are prone to sore throat in the colder months, make a big batch of this every winter: as soon as you feel a tickle in your throat you can get yourself a hot steaming cup and avoid getting a full-on cold and raspy throat.

Add any spices you like, such as allspice, clove, or star anise. You can also include orange peel: simply chop the peel of your (organic!) oranges and let dry fully before adding.

Stir in some lemon and honey if you like the flavors. Lemon has some antimicrobial action, and the sour and sweet flavors both stimulate the flow of healthy mucus, which fights infection.

You can also add a bit of butter, ghee, or coconut oil: less than ½ teaspoon per cup of hot tea. The medium-chain fatty acids (MCFAs) in these oils are topically antimicrobial and add a nice "coating" quality to the drink.

1 cup marshmallow root
½ cup dried ginger
¼ cup dried cinnamon bark
¼ cup dried licorice root

1. In a small bowl, mix together all the herbs. Store in an airtight container.
2. Make a decoction: Measure 2 to 4 tablespoons of herbs per quart of water and place in a lidded pot over high heat. Add the water and cover the pot. Bring to a boil, reduce the heat, and simmer for 1 hour.
3. To enhance the soothing effects of the mucilaginous herbs in this blend, cool the tea fully after decoction, then continue to cool for 1 to 2 more hours. Strain, and reheat before drinking.
4. Drink liberally throughout the day.

HERBAL GARGLE

Makes 16 fluid ounces (enough for several gargles)

Sage is an aromatic astringent, and it specifically kills rhinovirus: a virus that causes many colds. Combining it with vinegar and salt enhances these properties. If you have a dry sore throat, you may want to follow this with a nice cup of marshmallow tea.

8 fluid ounces water
2 tablespoons dried sage leaf
8 fluid ounces apple cider vinegar
3 teaspoons salt

1. In a small pot over high heat, bring the water to a boil. Remove it from the heat and add the sage. Cover tightly and let infuse for 20 minutes.
2. Strain the liquid into a pint-size mason jar.
3. Add the vinegar and salt, cover the jar, and shake well.
4. Pour off 1 fluid ounce or so and gargle with it for 2 to 3 minutes. Rinse your mouth out with water afterward—the vinegar's acidity can wear down tooth enamel if left in place.
5. Repeat 3 to 5 times per day.

THROAT~SOOTHING TEA

1 teaspoon Canadian fleabane leaves
1 teaspoon slippery elm bark
1 teaspoon echinacea root
2 cups boiling water

1. Combine the herbs in a nonmetallic container and cover with the boiling water; steep for 20 to 30 minutes; strain.
2. Take up to two cups per day, warm.

FRUITY GARGLE

1 tablespoon elderberry fruit juice
1 tablespoon sumac extract
1 teaspoon echinacea root extract

1. Combine the above ingredients and gargle, as needed.

SWEET COUGH DROPS

1 teaspoon goldenrod leaves
1 teaspoon wild cherry bark
1 teaspoon licorice root
1 teaspoon yerba sante leaves
1 teaspoon slippery elm bark
2 cups water
3 cups sugar
3 tablespoons corn syrup

1. Place the above herbs in a pan and cover with the water. Bring the mixture to a boil and boil for 20 minutes.
2. Remove from the heat and cool. Strain the solution and add the sugar and the corn syrup.
3. Place back on the heat, bring to a boil, then reduce heat to medium. Cook until the mixture reaches 300°F (hard-crack stage).
4. Pour the syrup onto a large, buttered baking sheet; cool, then break into one-inch pieces.
5. Use as you would any cough drop.

Sprains and Strains

A sprain occurs when a ligament is severely wrenched, while a strain is a tearing and overstretching of muscle fibers. The same injuries that can cause a sprain can cause a strain as well. The difference is that a sprain involves ligaments and tendons, while a strain involves muscles. Sprains and strains are very common and can cause pain, swelling, bruising, and inflammation. Movement in the affected area is often limited because of the pain and/or swelling.

Most sprains and strains may heal without complications. But more severe injuries can become chronic, develop scar tissue, limit motion, and ultimately cause problems in surrounding tissues, nerves, vessels, and organs.

Relevant tissue states: heat (inflammation), tension and/or laxity
Relevant herbal actions: anti-inflammatory, circulatory stimulant, connective tissue lubricant, lymphatic, nerve tropho-restorative, vulnerary

Herbal Allies

- Big Sagebrush
- Bilberry
- Black Cohosh
- Black Currant
- Cinnamon essential oil
- Gingko Biloba
- Ginger
- Ginseng
- Goldenrod leaf and flower
- Gotu Kola
- Horsetail
- Kelp
- Licorice
- Marshmallow
- Meadowsweet flower
- Peppermint essential oil
- Raspberry
- Self-heal leaf and flower
- Solomon's seal root
- St. John's wort leaf and flower
- Valerian
- White willow
- Wintergreen
- Yerba Mansa

The pain of an injured joint is your body speaking a warning to you. Heed it! Don't let a minor strain become a serious sprain. Rest the joint—but don't immobilize it; gentle movement allows blood to move through the injury site and speeds healing. Drink some bone broth (see Build-Up Broth), eat some seaweed, and work with herbs to reduce inflammation, improve blood exchange, and restore the connective tissues (tendons, ligaments, fascia).

One of the best methods for healing a sprain is alternating hot and cold compresses or baths. Heat exposure brings in fresh blood, while cold constricts the vessels and squeezes out stuck fluids. Alternate between 3 minutes of hot and 30 seconds of cold. Go back and forth a few times, and always finish with hot to bring fresh, healthy circulation to the area.

SOFT TISSUE INJURY LINIMENT

Makes about 8 fluid ounces (100+ applications, 30-day supply)

3 fluid ounces ginger-infused oil
2 fluid ounces Solomon's seal-infused oil or tincture of Solomon's seal
1 fluid ounce tincture of St. John's wort
1 fluid ounce tincture of self-heal
1 fluid ounce tincture of meadowsweet
40 drops peppermint essential oil
40 drops cinnamon essential oil

1.In a small bottle, combine the infused oils, tinctures, and essential oils. Cap the bottle and label it, including Shake well before each use.
2.Hold your palm over the bottle's mouth and tilt to deposit a small amount in your palm. Rub between your hands to warm the treatment, then apply to the painful joints.
3.Massage the oil into the joints until your hands no longer feel oily. Really work the liniment into the tissue.
4.Repeat the application 3 to 5 times per day. More is better!

TOPICAL PAIN RELIEF

20 drops yerba mansa tincture
4 ounces wintergreen oil
1 pound petroleum jelly

1. Thoroughly mix the above herbs with the petroleum jelly.
2. Use as an ointment to relieve muscle pain.

QUICK~ACTING PAIN RELIEF TEA

2 teaspoons black cohosh root
1 tablespoon ginseng root
2 cups water

1. Place the above herbs in a pan and cover with the water; bring to a boil; reduce heat and simmer for 30 minutes; cool and strain.
2. Take two to three tablespoons, up to six times a day.

SWEET RELIEF TEA

1 tablespoon raspberry leaves
1 teaspoon white willow bark
2 cups boiling water

1. Combine the above herbs and cover with the boiling water; steep for 30 minutes; strain.
2. Take as needed.

Stress

Increased heart rate, elevated blood pressure, muscle tension, irritability, depression, stomachache, and indigestion are all signs of stress. To many people, stress means emotional stress. But stress can also be physical (such as the injuries that occur because of a car accident or surgery) and biochemical (including exposure to pesticides or pollution and even poor nutrition). These (and other causes) make the body produce increased amounts of adrenaline. This is how the body copes with stress. But the adrenaline release also causes the heart rate to increase, blood pressure to rise, and muscles to tense.

A host of conditions can develop when the body is subjected to prolonged stress. These include an increased rate of aging, reduced resistance to infection, weakened immune function (which, in turn, can lead to other conditions such as chronic fatigue syndrome), and hormone overproduction (which can lead to adrenal fatigue).
The best tool to fight off the effects of stress is a well-balanced diet and lifestyle.

Relevant tissue states: heat (agitation), tension
Relevant herbal actions: adaptogen, nervine, relaxant, sedative

Herbal Allies

- Ashwagandha root
- Betony leaf and flower
- Catnip leaf and flower
- Chamomile flower
- Elderflower
- Ginger
- Goldenrod leaf and flower
- Hops
- Kava Kava
- Linden leaf and flower
- Peppermint
- Pleurisy
- Rose
- Sage leaf
- Skullcap
- St. John's wort leaf and flower
- Tulsi leaf
- Valerian

Everyone's stress is the same, and everyone's stress is different. We all have the same physiological response to stress—racing heart, shallow breathing, narrowed focus, heightened cortisol and blood sugar. But we react to potential stressors differently—something that bothers one person might roll right off another's back. Whatever is stressing you, herbs can help both as a short-term rescue in the immediate moment and in the long-term to build more "nerve reserve" and poise in the face of difficulties.

RESCUE ELIXIR

Makes 5 fluid ounces (40 to 80 doses)

When you need a quick respite from a hectic day, this is your best friend. This remedy works best if you can step away to a private space for a moment. Center yourself, breathe deeply for a few breaths, take your tincture, breathe a few more times, and return to the world. A little ritual goes a long way!

1 fluid ounce tincture of tulsi
1 fluid ounce tincture of betony
½ fluid ounce tincture of catnip
½ fluid ounce tincture of chamomile
½ fluid ounce tincture of elderflower
½ fluid ounce tincture of rose
¼ fluid ounce tincture of goldenrod
¼ fluid ounce tincture of sage
½ fluid ounce honey

1.In a small bottle, combine the tinctures and honey. Cap the bottle and label it.
2.Take 2 to 4 drops whenever needed.

SOOTHE UP! TEA

Makes 3¾ cups dried herb mix (enough for 22 to 30 quarts of tea)
This is the perfect mixture for those days when you feel like everything is falling down all around you: just take a moment, make a cup, drink it as deliberately as you can, and let the warmth and relaxation move through you.
If your stress manifests with a feeling of heaviness and downtrodden exhaustion, include ¼ cup of dried goldenrod and/or sage.
If it shows up as digestive upsets, include ¼ cup of dried chamomile and/or catnip.
Drink a quart or more every day.

1 cup dried betony leaf and flower
1 cup dried tulsi leaf
½ cup dried linden leaf and flower
½ cup dried rose petals
½ cup dried elderflower
¼ cup dried St. John's wort leaf and flower (see Tip)

1.In a medium bowl, mix together all the herbs. Store in an airtight container.
2.Make a hot infusion: Prepare a kettle of boiling water. Measure 2 to 3 tablespoons of herbs per quart of water and place in a mason jar or French press. Pour in the boiling water, cover, and steep for 20 minutes or until cool enough to drink.

TIP: Omit the St. John's wort if you are concurrently taking pharmaceuticals.

NERVE~SOOTHING TEA

1 teaspoon betony leaves
1 teaspoon kava kava root
1 teaspoon hops
1 teaspoon dried skullcap
1 cup boiling water
1. Combine the above herbs in a nonmetallic container.
2. Put two teaspoons of the mixture in another such container and cover with the boiling water; steep for 30 minutes; cool and strain.
3. Take one tablespoon at a time, as needed.

CALM DOWN TEA

1 teaspoon powdered ginger
1 teaspoon powdered valerian root
1 teaspoon powdered pleurisy root
2 cups boiling water

1. Combine the above herbs in a nonmetallic container and cover with the boiling water; steep for 30 minutes; cool and strain.
2. Take one tablespoon at a time, as needed, up to two cups a day.

SHAKE~IT~OFF TEA

1 to 2 teaspoons peppermint leaves
1 teaspoon valerian root
1 cup boiling water

1. Combine the above ingredients and cover with the boiling water; steep for 20 to 30 minutes; strain.
2. Drink up to one cup per day, as needed.

Wounds

Most wounds are caused by cuts, abrasions, or other physical injuries. Wounds should always be cleaned thoroughly to avoid an infection. The bleeding that often accompanies a wound can usually be stopped by applying pressure to the wound. Excessive bleeding, or injury to major arteries, requires immediate emergency medical care. If a wound turns red, swells, throbs, or is hot to the touch and contains pus, it is a sign of infection: please contact a medical professional immediately in this case.

Relevant tissue states: heat (inflammation)
Relevant herbal actions: antimicrobial, astringent, emollient, lymphatic, vulnerary

Herbal Allies

- Calendula flower
- Chamomile flower
- Goldenrod leaf and flower
- Kelp
- Marshmallow
- Pine
- Plantain leaf
- Rose
- Self-heal leaf and flower
- St. John's wort leaf and flower
- Yarrow leaf and flower

When working with a cut, scrape, abrasion, or other open wound, it's important to always follow the same order of operations:

Stop the bleeding. Direct application of pressure is usually the best way to accomplish this.

Clean the wound. Any particulate or foreign matter must be completely washed out of the wound or it will slow healing and allow infection to take root. A wound wash or soak with astringent, antimicrobial herbs is very effective for this stage.

Prevent or manage infection. Wound washes and soaks are also good here. Herb-infused honeys are extremely effective for this stage, serving both to disinfect and encourage healing. (Don't put tinctures directly into wounds unless you have no other option; even then, dilute them at 1 part tincture to 5 parts purified water, because alcohol inhibits cell growth.)

Encourage healing. Herb-infused honeys, poultices, compresses, and baths are all appropriate for open wounds. Once the wound closes (or if it was never very deep to begin with), you can transition to a salve. Choose herbs that are vulnerary, lymphatic (to drain blisters), and—especially in later stages—softening or emollient (to prevent scarring).

WOUND WASH

Makes 3 cups dried herb mix (enough for 10 to 20 quarts of wound wash)

If you're in a hurry, a simple wash with rose water or nonalcoholic witch hazel extract is very effective during the cleaning stage. After that, transition to soaks and compresses with a formula like this. In the later stages of wound healing, you may want to add ½ cup dried marshmallow or kelp for their emollient effects.

1. In a medium bowl, mix together all the herbs. Store in an airtight container.
2. Make a hot infusion: Prepare a kettle of boiling water. Measure 4 to 6 tablespoons of herbs per quart of water and place in a mason jar or French press. Pour in the boiling water, cover, and steep for 20 minutes or until cool.
3. Stir in 1 teaspoon of salt for each quart of infusion you've made.
4. Soak the wounded part, or apply a compress over the affected area.
5. Repeat as frequently as you can, at least 3 times per day.

PINE RESIN SALVE

Makes 8 ounces (40-day supply)

Pine resin salve is the best choice for wounds that have closed or were never very deep. You can work with the resin of other conifers, too. Resin can be harvested directly from the trees—you'll find whitish globs of it along the trunk where branches were lost. Leave enough on the tree to keep the wound sealed—this resin is how the tree forms a scab!
It will probably have bits of bark, dirt, insect parts, etc., stuck in it—don't worry: you'll filter that out during processing.
After gathering resin, use a bit of oil to wash your hands—soap and water won't work. Just drop a bit of any liquid oil you have handy into your hands and scrub as if it were soap. The resin will soften and separate from your skin. Then you can use soap and hot water to wash it away.
You can use plain oil for infusing your resin but starting with an herb-infused oil means you get the good actions of all these herbs, instead of just those the resin contributes.

6 to 8 ounces pine resin or another conifer resin
8 fluid ounces total calendula-infused oil, goldenrod-infused oil, and/or plantain-infused oil
1 ounce beeswax, chopped or grated, plus more as needed

1. In a small pan over low heat, combine the resin and infused oil and heat gently, stirring frequently. The resin will soften and dissolve, infusing the oil with its virtues.

2.Pour this warm oil through a few layers of cheesecloth. Wrap the mass that remains and squeeze it to extract as much oil as possible.

3.Prepare a salve using this resin-infused oil (see here for complete instructions).

4.Apply to the wound several times a day, using fresh, neat bandages each time.

TOPICAL APPLICATION FOR ABRASIONS

1 teaspoon white pine inner bark
1 teaspoon wild cherry bark
1 teaspoon wild plum root
2 cups water

1. Combine the above herbs in a pan and cover with the water.
2. Bring to a boil and boil until the bark and roots are soft.
3. Cool and strain.
4. To use, soak a clean (preferably sterilized) cloth in the solution and apply to the affected area.

TOPICAL WASH FOR CUTS

1 teaspoon pleurisy root
1 teaspoon ginseng root
2 cups water

1. Combine the above herbs in a pan and cover with the water; bring to a boil and boil for 20 to 30 minutes; strain.
2. Apply topically, as needed.

Conclusion

I hope you have enjoyed reading this book as much as I've enjoyed writing it, and I hope it will accompany you in your ongoing journey to the discovery of Native American herbs and their medicinal uses.

If you found this book useful and are feeling generous, please take the time to leave a short review on Amazon so that other may enjoy this guide as well.

I leave you with good wishes and hopefully a better knowledge of the plants around us and their amazing powers.

Made in the USA
Monee, IL
26 April 2021